Sylvia Klein Olkin has a Masters degree in Education/Eastern Studies and has taught yoga classes at many different levels since 1975. She has appeared on numerous talk shows as well as panel discussions on yoga and meditation.

Joy,

Sylvia Klein Olkin

Sylvia Klein Olkin

Positive Pregnancy
through
Yoga

A SPECTRUM BOOK

Prentice-Hall, Inc., Englewood Cliffs, N.J. 07632

Library of Congress Cataloging in Publication Data

Olkin, Sylvia Klein.
   Positive pregnancy through yoga.

   (A Spectrum Book)
   Bibliography: p.
   Includes index.
   1. Pregnancy.   2. Prenatal care.   3. Yoga, Hatha.
4. Exercise for women.   I. Title.
RG558.7.O43   618.2'4   81-2582
ISBN 0-13-687632-3
ISBN 0-13-687624-2 (pbk.)   AACR2

This Spectrum Book is available to businesses and organizations at a special discount when ordered in large quantities. For information, contact Prentice-Hall, Inc., General Book Marketing, Special Sales Division, Englewood Cliffs, N.J. 07632.

10   9   8   7   6   5   4   3   2   1

Editorial/production supervision
and interior design by Kimberly Mazur
Page layout by Marie Alexander and Mary Greey
Cover design by Judith Leeds
Manufacturing buyer: Cathie Lenard

All line drawings by Sandra Lucas, except pages
11, 97, and 128 by Pete Smith.
All photos by Edmund J. Burke, except on page 201
by David Howe, bottom of 216 by Naomi Howe, and top
of 216 by Deborah Beckwith.

Prentice-Hall International, Inc., *London*
Prentice-Hall of Australia Pty. Limited, *Sydney*
Prentice-Hall of Canada, Ltd., *Toronto*
Prentice-Hall of India Private Limited, *New Delhi*
Prentice-Hall of Japan, Inc., *Tokyo*
Prentice-Hall of Southeast Asia Pte. Ltd., *Singapore*
Whitehall Books Limited, *Wellington, New Zealand*

To my husband, Bob,
my sons, Mathew and Michael,
my parents, Nora and Meyer Klein,
my Yoga teachers, Bob and Thelma Peck,
and my family for their continual love, enthusiasm and support

to Naomi, David, and Dana Howe,
for giving so generously of their
time, talent, ideas, and love.

Contents

LABOR AND BIRTH

Foreword

For over twenty-five years I have practiced obstetrics and gynecology and have noticed that women desire to be more informed and active participants in their pregnancies. Sylvia Klein Olkin's book, *Positive Pregnancy Through Yoga,* is a fascinating and practical approach to the preparation for pregnancy, labor, and delivery.

Sylvia Klein Olkin has been interested in yoga for many years and has taught at a variety of places from Connecticut College to the local YMCA. She has combined her own personal experience with her knowledge of yoga to develop special classes for the management of prepared childbirth. I have known Sylvia for a number of years, and it has been a pleasure to see the expertise and feeling she brings to the woman who is trying to prepare herself for pregnancy, labor, and delivery. Sylvia has researched her information well and has sought expert advice on the subjects she has included in her book.

Positive Pregnancy Through Yoga is a book I would recommend to all my patients as a useful way to help themselves have a happy and successful childbearing experience.

Frank J. Carter, M.D.
President of the Staff
Senior, Department of OB/GYN
Wm. W. Backus Hospital
Norwich, Connecticut
Assistant Clinical Professor
School of Nursing, Yale University

Preface

One sunny spring morning four years ago, I walked into my wood-paneled yoga classroom and was greeted by an enthusiastic group of students. In this group were three women, all in different stages of pregnancy. Two had been sent by their doctors to learn how to relax; the third was a woman I knew quite well. She had attended my yoga classes during the preceding year, although I had not seen her for several months. She said that she wanted to continue her study of yoga all during the time she was expecting her first child. She felt that yogic practice would help her more fully to experience and enjoy the waiting months.

A normal yoga program would have many limitations for these three mothers-to-be. Several of the basic yogic positions or asanas are *not* wise to practice during pregnancy. I soon realized that expectant mothers needed a special class of their own.

The following summer, I began the research that has evolved into this book. At that time, I read many books and talked with numerous doctors, nurses, midwives, a psychologist, a professor of obstetrical nursing, and many, many pregnant women. I began to understand which parts of the pregnant body needed to be especially prepared for birth, as well as the necessity of relaxation skills for a positive birth experience; more important, I began to explore the mental space of pregnancy.

I will never forget teaching my first "Yoga for the Mother-to-Be" class. After all the research, thinking, wondering, and talking, here I was facing fifteen real live pregnant women!

The room was very small, and the mats on which we would stretch were crammed in, literally, wall to wall. As I was about to begin, I looked around at the faces of all my students. They were not quite sure what to expect and, to a certain extent, neither was I.

I happened to look around the room for a second time and this time I could have sworn that I saw another set of eyes, tiny eyes, looking back at me! It was at that moment that the duality of pregnancy became very real to me. I was engulfed with a feeling of sheer panic. Was I prepared? Would all fifteen women feel better after the class had ended? Were the asanas as safe and useful in real life as I thought them to be? With these questions and others racing through my mind, I quickly did some yogic abdominal breathing and plunged in. The deep breathing turned the panic into a calmness that could be shared by all in the class as I began. I have been teaching prenatal yoga ever since.

It is a continually rewarding experience to spend time and share space with pregnant women. There is a special feeling . . . a special energy . . . a special love in these groups. Much of the most useful information in this book was discovered or created in my prenatal classes. The asanas, breathing exercises, concentrations, and meditations have been "people–tested" and proven safe and effective, producing positive and lasting results. Many of the most useful ideas found here were contributed by my students.

In order for you to use this book more easily, soften the binding by opening the book to the center and then placing the front and back covers together. With your fingers, work up and down the binding so that it becomes softer. Once you have done this, the book should stay open and flat without any difficulty.

I have tried to make this book as personal as possible in order to duplicate the personal attention my students receive while attending my classes.

I sincerely hope that the yogic program contained in this book helps you to harmonize your inner and outer worlds, thereby enabling you to enjoy and experience pregnancy and motherhood more fully.

Yours in peace,
Sylvia

ACKNOWLEDGMENTS

The creation, development, and completion of this book would not have been possible without the generous efforts of a special group of people. My sincere thanks to:

Bob and Thelma Peck, for making me aware of the seed that developed into this book, and for being yoga teachers who continually share their time, love, and enthusiasm for life.

Ed Burke, for his time, effort, and photographic talent.

Dr. Frank Carter, for his practical and helpful medical advice.

Beth Carter, for her editorial assistance and ideas.

Frederick Leboyer, for his enlightening correspondence on "inner bonding."

Helaine Klein Ronen, for editing and typing the original proposal for this book.

Heidi Wolfman and the staff of the Norwich YMCA, for launching my yoga teaching career and encouraging the development of new yoga courses.

Patricia Donohue, clinical dietician, for her time, effort, and knowledge devoted to the nutrition chapter.

Amy Dunion, R.N., certified childbirth educator, for her information on the Lamaze childbirth breathing program.

Linda Green, R.N., M.S., for her helpful research on the physiology of pregnancy and birth.

Jan Lindberg, herbologist, for his research on herbs and pregnancy.

Ann McNamara, La Leche League leader, for her helpful information on breastfeeding.

Bill McNamara and Bob Crooks, for their expert instruction on massage.

Arlene Belzer, for her editorial advice.

Theresa Ammirati, for proofreading the manuscript and for her editorial assistance.

Chris Boezeman, for her cheerful attitude and expert manuscript typing.

The Monday and Tuesday night meditation classes, for their encouragement and energy.

Sandy Lucas, for her continual creativity used to illustrate what I couldn't explain.

Peter H. Smith, for his innate artistic talent and positive attitude.

Peg and Ed Lambright, for their time and concern printing the illustrative photographs.

Barbara Smith, bread-making teacher, for her herb bread recipes.

Marjorie Blizard, for the original conception of the Complimentary Proteins illustrations.

Lynne Lumsden, my acquisitions editor at Prentice-Hall, for believing in *Positive Pregnancy through Yoga.*

Kim Mazur, my production editor at Prentice-Hall, for her cooperation, enthusiasm, accuracy, and faith.

My parents and entire family, for their continual support and goodwill for the duration of this project.

And most of all to my students, for their time, enthusiasm, ideas, and lots and lots of love.

I wish you all:

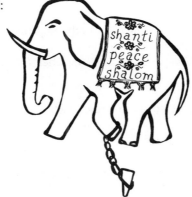

Part I
Positive Pregnancy

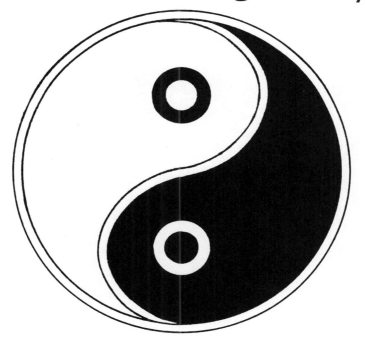

"Yin-Yang," Chinese symbol of duality in Nature

One

Life with a Yogic Slant

Imagine that you are looking at a still photograph of a lovely tropical scene. In your mind's eye, see the palm trees, the white sandy beach, the varied, colorful flowers, vines and trees. Embellish this mental picture with a deep blue cloudless sky, the blue-green waters of a calm lagoon bathed in golden sunshine. See the variety of people on the beach: two small children digging in the sand, a young man reading, an older couple playing cards, two teenagers lazily swimming in the calm water. A small sailboat is on the horizon and its inhabitants are waving to the young man on the beach. Try to make this scene as real as you can.

Now let's make this scene more real and exciting by turning it into a moving picture. Mentally see the palm trees blowing and bending lazily in the breeze as the people begin to move about doing their own activities. See the children constructing a large sand city. They have already built the smaller buildings and are building the main castle with a high elaborate moat. One child is going to get water in his bucket to fill in the moat around the castle. Hear the sounds of the warm calm water lapping lazily onto the beach as the birds' chirping blends with the sounds of unfinished conversations on the beach. Several new people are coming onto the beach; mentally see who they are and what they are doing. Try to make yourself a part of this moving picture by imagining how you would feel if you were in this very beautiful scene. Imagine how the scene would smell, sound, and feel to you.

You may be wondering after all this imaginary work what the connection is between these scenes and the study of yoga. The connection is really quite simple. Life without yoga can be compared to a still photograph of a place. You will see all the parts of the scene, but you will miss the action. You can easily be contented with this still view of life, but there really is more to life for you to explore and experience. The discipline of yoga can enable you to fully experience and enjoy the various levels of your life. By learning more about how you function—your brain and your body—you will learn to heighten your senses, thereby deepening your daily experiences. You will, in essence, become more alive. It may seem illogical to you for a "discipline" to give you enjoyment and pleasure. Usually people think of "discipline" as punishment or something to be avoided at all costs. We discipline our children when they exhibit unacceptable behavior. From a yogic point of view, "discipline" is the application of the yogic rules and exercises to all aspects of your life. By merely integrating yogic practices into your daily routine, you will begin to notice things about yourself that you were not aware of before. When you begin to notice things about yourself, you begin to notice new things about people and the outside world as well. With the excitement, anxiety, and expectancy of a new baby growing inside you, the benefits to be derived from practicing yoga are varied and large.

Use your imagination once again and come with me to one of my "Yoga for the Mother-to-Be" classes. It is the first class of an eight-week series, and the new students are walking down the brightly lit corridor carrying their blankets, pillows, and purses, looking for the meeting room. Some of the women are walking with the pregnancy waddle of the later months; some are just beginning to show. Once my new students have found the room and gotten settled on their mats, lively conversation inevitably begins. If you listen closely, you can hear someone asking, "When are you due?" or "How much weight have you gained so far?" or "You have a backache, too?"

There is a special feeling in this room. A feeling of anticipation, of expectancy, of heightened energy. Each woman is here to prepare herself for a very important event: the birth of her baby, and of a new consciousness, into the world. She wants to be in good physical, mental, and emotional shape in order to enhance her birthing experience. I am sure you want these same things too.

When I begin the class with each woman introducing herself and indicating her due date, it is fun to see which women will be having their babies at the same time of year. Next comes the barrage of questions; there are always so many on the first evening of class. "What kind of exercises should I *not* be doing?" "Can I continue to jog?" "What is a well balanced diet anyhow?" "What does yoga have to do with having a baby?" Maybe you have one to ask. This is only a brief sampling of the many questions asked and answered during this class session. These pregnant women want simple answers and remedies to the everyday complaints or experiences of pregnancy. They want the answers fast, for their time is limited and they have a lot to learn before their babies arrive.

I explain that an ancient system of self-discipline has the answers for which they have been searching. At this point someone usually asks, "What is yoga?" You may be curious about this question as well. The best way to explain yoga is to say that it is a highly scientific system for self-improvement and self-knowledge. The word "yoga" is from an ancient Indian language called Sanskrit. It derives from a verbal root "yuk" which literally means to "yoke, join together, or unite." The yogic system, if practiced correctly, can allow the student to experience the union of the mind and the body and eventually union with the Universal Spirit. The term "hatha," which describes the physical aspect of yoga, literally means sun (ha) and moon (tha). This is symbolic of the warm and cool aspects of each individual that can be integrated by the practice of physical yoga. This integration can lead to an even flow of energy through the body's channels as well as increased good health. Mental and physical harmony are the goals achieved by consistent practice. By combining the physical system with some forms of controlled breathing, relaxation and/or meditation, you can contribute to your own development and perfection both physically and spiritually.

After this rather deep philosophical explanation of hatha yoga and how it works, a student often asks, "But what does all that stuff have to do with having a baby?" That is a very valid question, and if you think about the foregoing information for a moment, you may begin to have a glimmer of what yoga is all about. Remember that the word yoga means union. When you are pregnant, it is the only time in your life that you are experiencing a daily physical union with another being. Your body and that of the baby are continually interconnected. The baby is dependent on you all during its development. Thus you are actually experiencing a form of union or yoga while you are pregnant. It is a very different form from what is generally described in the ancient yogic writings, but it is one level of yoga nonetheless. Since you are in such a close relationship with your future child, if you take the time to learn control of your body and your mind while you are pregnant, it is exceedingly beneficial for the baby growing within. Your baby is extremely sensitive to your ups and downs.

Finally, it is time to stretch into our first yoga asana. Here is another Sanskrit word which describes the special kind of movements which are the cornerstone of a physical yoga program. *Asana* is a position which is easy and comfortable as well as firm. This means going into a stretch, keeping your mind on the feelings it is giving you and holding it for as long as is comfortable. You may want to imagine that you are a member of this imaginary class right now and try your first yoga asana with us. Read these directions over twice before you try out this simple arm stretch. It is very important for inner centering that you keep your eyes closed and feel your body move.

Simple Arm Stretch

- Lift your arms slowly up above your head.
- Feel your arm muscles working as you move.
- Clasp your hands, turn the palms toward the ceiling, and stretch.
- Breathe normally as you mentally feel your arms stretch and your rib cage move up.
- Hold for as long as is comfortable and then slowly float the arms down to your sides.

Once your arms return to your sides, if you observe yourself carefully, you will find that your body will automatically take a breath. Next it is time to learn to take a deep yogic abdominal breath. Here again there is the mental concentration on every bodily movement as we all deep breathe together.

Yogic Abdominal Breath

- Place your hands on the baby area.
- Relax the tummy.
- Inhale through the nose and move the tummy (baby) forward.
- Immediately exhale through the nose and move the tummy (baby) back.
- Repeat this breath again.

This breath will balance out the stretch as well as wash carbon dioxide from your muscles so you do not ache later.

This deep breath is followed by many new and interesting stretches as the prenatal physical program unfolds. Finally time has slipped away and the end of class is nearing. After all the new bends and stretches of the asana program, most students are only too glad to get into a comfortable position and relax their minds and bodies completely for several minutes. Once the complete relaxation is completed and the students are beginning to move again, the earlier restlessness is gone, replaced by an inner calm. Many new yoga students have commented that they really do not fully understand life with a yogic slant, but they know it feels terrific.

You can join this group of students by participating in my prenatal classes via this book. If you take some private time each day to come into my classroom, your senses will be heightened, your worries eased, and your total enjoyment of life increased. Yoga will not eliminate trouble from your life, but it will help you see from a new perspective so that you can live life to the fullest at this very exciting time. The joy in life is there for the taking. It is double when you are pregnant! There is joy in little things which you may have missed before. Taking a deep breath and feeling the extra vitality in your body feels wonderful. Maybe your baby will kick and say "thank-you" for the extra boost of energy received. Have you ever closed your eyes and *really* tasted a raisin? Try it, you may be very surprised. From a yogic point of view, life is to be enjoyed and experienced to the fullest. There is so much to see, taste, feel, hear, and know. Life is full of movement, vitality, and change just as in a moving picture. Don't miss all the action by not paying attention to it while you think or worry about what could happen or what happened ten years ago. Once you learn to quiet your mind and tune into your body and baby, you can truly begin to experience and enjoy the beautiful world in which we live.

Two
Conscious Breathing: Key to Relaxation

Pregnancy is a special time to share consciously with your unborn child. That idea is appealing, but you may be wondering *how* you can go about doing that. The answer is a very simple one: through your breathing. Focusing all your attention on your child and on the natural breathing process of your body for only a few minutes a day will give you such amazing results, I am sure you will be happily surprised. After introducing abdominal or "Rock-the-Baby" breathing to my students in their very first prenatal yoga class, I usually instruct the women to try the breathing out at red lights, while waiting in line at the supermarket, during television commercials, etc. It is always fun to hear the reaction to this type of breathing during the second class. Some comments I have heard are: "It's amazing how quickly it works." "I was getting a headache, then I took five Rock-the-Baby breaths and the head-ache just disappeared." "I couldn't get back to sleep in the middle of the night after my third trip to the bathroom, and the breathing worked like a charm."

What is the deep dark secret behind all these success stories? It is merely using the tummy or baby area while deep breathing and being totally conscious of each breath. Sounds simple? Well, it is and it is not. Invariably when I first describe abdominal breathing, one or two women say that this technique is the opposite of the way they normally breathe. This is perfectly correct. However, it is much easier to learn yogic abdominal breathing during preg-nancy, with the added advantage of the prominent tummy.

This chapter contains a variety of breathing exercises which will naturally ease you over some of the rougher times of your pregnancy and move you very smoothly into motherhood. Try all the breathing techniques at least once to see which you prefer to use. Check the benefits, which vary widely, so that you will know when to use which breath.

A mandala is a geometric design used by many yoga students as a point of concentration. This mandala (Figure 2.1) has been especially created for your use to develop your outward concentration while practicing the breathing exercises (pranayamas). This practice will be most useful to you during labor and delivery. It can help you to breathe through your contractions with an outward focus. Try centering your awareness on the center of the mandala as you practice one of the many breathing exercises within this chapter.

Figure 2.1   Mandala for practicing breathing exercises: Keep your concentration on the center point as you breathe.

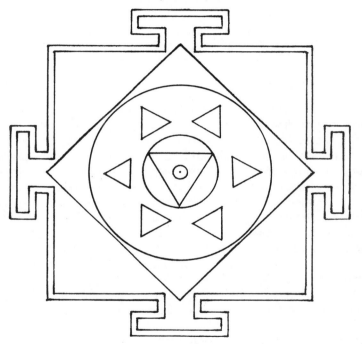

THE PHYSIOLOGY OF BREATHING

In order to take a really deep breath, you have to learn to relax and use your abdominal muscles. If you breathe with a tight tummy, you shrink your body's air capacity, thereby allowing your diaphragm and rib muscles to grow weak while leaving the blood hungry for oxygen. Breathing with a tight tummy also means more wear on the body; you have to take two to three shallow breaths to equal the amount of oxygen you take in with one deep abdominal breath.

Some basic knowledge of body physiology will help you understand the different processes which are involved when you take a yogic abdominal breath. The parts of your body which are most directly involved in the breathing process are the nose (through which the air travels), the trachea or windpipe (connecting link to the lungs) and the lungs (where oxygen is exchanged for carbon dioxide with each breath). The section of the body in which the heart and the lungs are located is called the thorax or the chest cavity. The neck is the upper part of the thorax, while the diaphragm (which is a thick muscle) forms the floor of the thorax. Below the thorax and the diaphragm is the abdominal area of your body, which contains the organs of digestion, reproduction, and excretion (Figure 2.2). When you consciously relax the abdominal muscles and inhale, the diaphragm moves downward, thereby increasing your lung capacity (see Figure 2.3). At the same time, there is a reduction of air pressure in the lungs, and fresh air comes into the lungs because of a vacuum-type pull. With the diaphragmatic downstroke, the interior organs of the abdomen receive a gentle massage which helps improve digestion and circulation. When exhaling, you need to slightly contract the abdominal wall. This will cause the diaphragm to return to a domed position pushing upward, which will expel the carbon dioxide from your lungs (see Figure 2.4).

Figures 2.2, 2.3, 2.4 (From left to right)   The thorax and abdominal areas of the body; Yogic Abdominal Breath during an inhalation; Yogic Abdominal Breath during an exhalation.

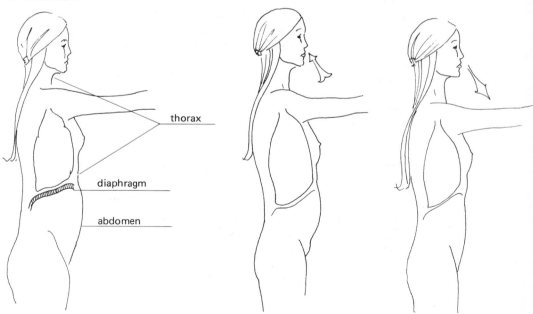

thorax

diaphragm

abdomen

SHALLOW BREATHING

Poor breathing habits can have very negative effects on your body. Upper chest breathing usually leads to illness of one sort or another which is often accompanied by mental depression. While you are carrying and nurturing a child, you must be aware of how you can best fulfill the needs of this new person. Learning to breathe abdominally can be one of the most positive steps you can take to insure the well–being of both yourself and your baby. Just as you are eating for two while you are pregnant, you are breathing for two as well.

BREATHING AND EMOTIONS

Have you ever noticed when you are going through a highly emotional time that your breathing is ragged and uneven, just as your emotions are? When you are feeling depressed, you may unconsciously lower your head and let your shoulders fall forward, thereby lessening your lung capacity. The more you cut down your lung capacity, the more depressed and irrational you will feel. The brain needs three times the amount of oxygen used by the rest of the body. No wonder you make very little sense when you are highly emotional!

The ancient yogis spent much time studying the effects of breathing on the physical and mental processes of the body. They concluded that learning to control the breath was one very important key to happiness in this life. That is why there is such a great emphasis on correct breathing in any physical yoga program. During pregnancy when blood volume increases up to 50 percent by the end of the nine months, correct deep abdominal breathing is even more important. It is important to remember that the full responsibility for your emotional state is in your hands, or perhaps "lungs" would be a more accurate description! You really can control your moods by using even, rhythmic, deep breathing methods as natural "uppers."

GUIDELINES FOR PRACTICING BREATHING

You may think the idea of "practicing breathing" is very strange since you have been breathing all your life without any guidelines. However, in order to derive the most benefit from the following exercises, certain rules need to be followed.

1. Check with your doctor or midwife before beginning a yoga breathing exercise program.

2. Use your nose for inhaling and exhaling, unless otherwise instructed. The nasal passages will clean, warm, and moisten the air before it enters your lungs and then your blood system.

3. Do not ever hold your breath during these breathing exercises. This would not be beneficial for your child.

4. You must learn to keep your awareness on either the baby or on your breath as you practice in order to obtain the desired results.

5. You must practice each breath at least five to ten times to receive the desired benefits. It is the repetition of the process with coordinated mental concentration that will cause you to either revitalize or calm down.

BREATHS TO BE USED DAILY

Yogic Abdominal Breath
or Rock-The-Baby Breath

This can be practiced in any sitting, standing, or lying down position.

Benefits:
- Consciously connects you to your future child
- Calms your nerves
- Enriches and purifies your blood and the baby's because of increased oxygen intake
- Increases resistance to colds and other respiratory conditions

Directions:
1. Sitting in a cross-legged position on your mat or comfortably in a chair, place your right hand on your tummy. Check to see that your head is up straight, your facial muscles are relaxed, and your back is as straight as is comfortable.

2. Exhale as completely as you can through your nose.

3. Relax your tummy muscles and begin to inhale through your nose sending the air directly to the baby area. You should feel the tummy move slightly forward. The shoulders should be perfectly still.

4. Once you have completely filled the tummy area, which should take about five seconds, begin to smoothly exhale. *Do not hold your breath.*

5. As you exhale, which should take about five to eight seconds, slightly contract the abdominal muscles until you have completed the exhalation.

6. The tummy moves forward as you inhale and backward as you exhale; hence the name "Rock-the-Baby" breath.

7. Keep your awareness on your breath coming in and rocking your baby forward and your breath going out and rocking the baby backward. Often you may find you can concentrate better with your eyes closed.

8. Repeat five to ten times and relax.

Cautions and Comments:

- Do not practice this breath too fast or you may feel dizzy.
- If you do feel dizzy, you are breathing too quickly. Slow down and the dizziness will disappear.
- As you practice you will find that you will be able to inhale and exhale for longer periods of time.
- The baby may start kicking in appreciation for the extra boost of energy you are giving it when you practice this exercise.
- Once you have mastered this breath, you do not have to keep your right hand on your tummy.
- Practice this exercise at red lights, while waiting to see the doctor, during T.V. commercials, or any time you have a spare moment.

Baby Breath

This is easiest to learn in a squatting position; once mastered, it can be practiced in any position.

Benefits:

- Mentally and physically prepares you to utilize the birth canal area of your body for your baby's birth
- Reminds you of the birth process on a daily basis
- Helps to keep your sexual muscles well toned
- Calms your nerves

Directions:

1. Stand up straight on your mat with your feet eight to ten inches apart.

2. Turn your feet out to the sides on a 45° angle. Stretch your arms straight out in front of your chest, palms down.

3. Slowly go down into a regular squatting position, either on your toes or on flat feet. You may want to have a chair in front of you for support, if you have not mastered squatting.

4. Once you're in a squatting position, rest your hands on your knees or clasp them in front of you if you are not using a chair (Figure 2.5).

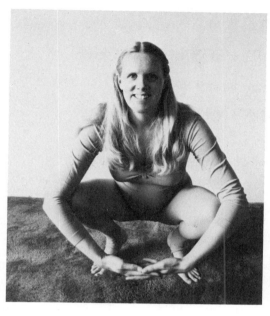

Figure 2.5 A squatting position for practicing "Baby Breath."

5. Relax all of your facial muscles. *Imagine* as you begin to inhale in the usual manner that you are inhaling through your navel directly to the baby. Your tummy will move slightly forward.

6. As you exhale *imagine* that you are exhaling through the birth canal as you push down and forward slightly by using your vaginal muscles. *Imagine* that the breath is taking the same route which your baby will take when it is being born.

7. You may feel the bottom of your tummy contracting as you exhale and this is fine.

8. Repeat five to ten times and relax.

Cautions and Comments:
• Do not be discouraged if it takes you a while to learn this breath. The effort will surely be worth it!

• Do not push down too hard; it is a very subtle movement.

• One student commented on this breath: "My doctor and nurse were amazed at how well I was able to push. I really feel that the idea of 'Baby Breath' [exhaling through the birth canal] made this part of delivery easy."

- Practicing this breath will help to facilitate and possibly shorten your pushing time when you are having your baby.
- Practice it between asanas, while driving, etc.

BREATHS TO REMEDY HEADACHES

Alternate Nostril Breath

This breath should only be practiced in a sitting position

Benefits:
- Calms both your body and your mind
- Helps to overcome negative feelings such as fear, worry, and anxiety
- Helps to relieve sinus conditions
- Strengthens your nervous system
- Can minimize and/or eliminate headaches and insomnia
- Can help to keep blood pressure at normal levels
- Makes you feel very peaceful and serene

Directions:
1. Sitting cross-legged on your mat or comfortably in a chair, with your back and head up straight, bring your right palm in front of your face.
2. Bend the second and third fingers on your right hand. Lightly close off the left nostril with your fourth and fifth fingers. Leave the right nostril open (Figure 2.6).
3. Relax your facial muscles and close your eyes. Begin inhaling smoothly and evenly on the right using a "Rock-the-Baby" breath. When you have inhaled as fully as you can through the right nostril without straining, close it off with your thumb.
4. Open the left nostril by moving your fourth finger and exhale completely on the left side (Figure 2.7). The exhalation will usually be longer than the inhalation. Once the exhalation is completed, close off the left side again and begin to inhale on the right. Repeat this same procedure for five breaths. (Breathe in right and out left, five times.)
5. After the fifth breath, change the sequence by inhaling on the left and exhaling on the right for five breaths.
6. After completing ten rounds or breaths, rest your hands in your lap, keep your eyes closed, and look inside to see how you feel.

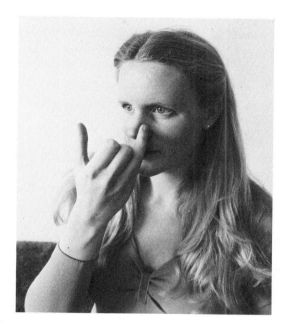

Figure 2.6 Alternate Nostril Breath with the left nostril closed.

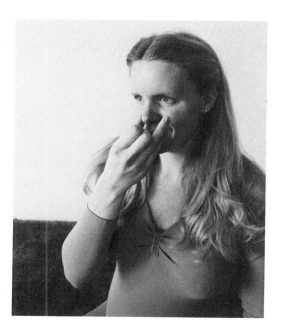

Figure 2.7 Alternate Nostril Breath with the right nostril closed.

Cautions and Comments:

- Breathe evenly, quietly, and without strain although one nostril may be more open than the other. If you feel you are not inhaling enough, use your mouth for part of the inhalation. Exhale through your nose.
- Follow the breath mentally with each inhalation and exhalation.
- As soon as you feel the beginning of a headache, this is an excellent technique to use to eliminate the situation.
- Do not hold your breath while practicing this exercise.
- This breath is often called the sun/moon breath since, according to yoga, it is believed that one nostril is active or positive (sun) while the other is passive and negative (moon). Alternate nostril breathing restores equilibrium to the body by balancing the opposite currents in the body.
- Practice this breath for ten rounds before meditating.

BREATHS FOR SPECIFIC PURPOSES

Anti Insomnia Breath

This can be practiced lying on your left side in bed.

Benefits:

- Helps to eliminate insomnia
- Strengthens your breathing mechanism
- Calms and slows you down without harmful drugs

Directions:

1. Lying on your left side in a comfortable position, close off your right nostril with your right thumb.
2. Close your eyes and inhale and exhale using only the left nostril. Use the "Rock-the-Baby" breath.
3. Do 15 smooth, slow inhalations and 15 even, complete exhalations.
4. As you are breathing, think, "Inhale 15," "Exhale 15"; "Inhale 14," "Exhale 14"; "Inhale 13," "Exhale 13"; etc.
5. It is very important to keep your mental concentration on counting the breaths. (This helps to bore you to sleep!)
6. When you have finished the breathing, place the right hand into a comfortable position and begin a complete mental relaxation (p. 155).
7. Begin by relaxing your facial muscles, then your neck, etc.
8. Let yourself fall off to sleep.

Cautions and Comments:
- If you are up in the middle of the night, it is often useful to have a hot glass of milk, read for 10–15 minutes, then go back to bed and do this breath.
- If you are left-handed, these directions must be reversed. For left-handed people the passive nostril is the right nostril.

Remember that your dominant or active nostril is the same as your dominant hand. Only using the dominant or active nostril for breathing will energize you. Only using the passive nostril for breathing will put you to sleep.

Energizing Single Nostril Breath

This can be practiced sitting up, standing, lying down.

Benefits:
- Energizes your body and your mind
- Increases alertness while eliminating fatigue
- Strengthens your breathing mechanism

Directions:
1. Arrange yourself in any comfortable position.
2. Close your left nostril with your right pointer finger.
3. Close your eyes and inhale and exhale on the right side only using the "Rock-the-Baby" breath. Do ten smooth, slow inhalations and ten even, complete exhalations.
4. As you inhale, think, "Inhale energy one." As you exhale, think, "Exhale tiredness one"; then continue, "Inhale energy two," "Exhale tiredness two," etc., until you reach ten. It is very important to keep your mental concentration on these thoughts.
.5. Let the right hand rest and keep the eyes closed as your breathing returns to normal upon completion of the ten rounds.
6. Within five to ten minutes you will begin to feel revitalized and renewed.

Cautions and Comments:
- Do not substitute this breath for sleep when your body is truly tired.
- If you are left-handed, these directions must be reversed. For left-handed people the dominant nostril is the left nostril.

Soft Sighing Breath

This can be practiced in any position.

Benefits
- Releases stored tensions and anxieties
- Flushes the lungs of wastes
- Refreshes and recharges the body
- Prepares the throat for mouth centered breathing in labor

Directions:
1. Arrange yourself in a comfortable position. Relax your facial muscles and close your eyes.
2. Inhale fully and smoothly using the "Rock-the-Baby" breath.
3. Exhale through the mouth allowing the air to touch the back of the throat. It should sound like a soft sighing "haa" sound.
4. When you are practicing this breath, imagine that you have just finished the job you like to do the least and you are sighing with relief now that it is over.
5. Repeat five to ten times and rest.

Cautions and Comments:
- Do not force the air out; merely let it come out naturally.
- Be dramatic when you practice this. If you do, many stored up tensions will disappear.
- Keep your mouth and throat as loose as you can when practicing.
- Do not be embarrassed if you make sounds. Sighing is one of the body's natural ways to release tensions.

CALMING BREATHS

Smooth Breath

This can be practiced in any position.

Benefits:
- Quiets, calms, relaxes and stabilizes the mind and body
- Develops excellent control of the breathing process
- Helps to ensure emotional balance

Directions:

1. Arrange yourself in a comfortable position. Relax your facial muscles.

2. Directing all your attention to your breathing, begin to inhale as in "Rock-the-Baby" breath. Make the inhalation as smooth as possible. Imagine the breath going down into the baby area and beginning to go around the baby.

3. As you begin to exhale, imagine the breath completing its circle around the baby and coming back up to your nose for exhalation.

4. Make sure that the change from inhalation to exhalation is as quiet and smooth as possible so as not to disturb the baby.

5. Practice five to ten of these breaths and then rest.

Cautions and Comments:

- This breath may seem difficult at first, but with practice it becomes very enjoyable.

- The control you can learn by practicing this breath will be very helpful to you during labor.

- Try not to pause between inhalations and exhalations. Make the transition as smooth as you can.

- Let your breath encircle your child with energy and vitality.

Mountain Breath

This should be practiced either sitting or standing.

Benefits:

- Calms your nervous system

- Expands the rib cage thereby increasing oxygen intake and improving lung capacity

- Tones the chest, abdomen and pelvic muscles

- Eliminates stitch in rib cage area often experienced in late pregnancy

- Improves digestion and elimination

Directions:

1. Stand up tall and straight on your mat with your feet facing forward about six to eight inches apart. Be sure your feet are evenly placed.

2. Place the palms of your hands together with your thumbs resting against your breastbone and the fingertips facing upwards.

3. Relax the tummy muscles and begin inhaling while you move your joined hands in front of your face and straight up as far as possible.

4. As you begin to exhale, separate your hands and sweep them out sideways, then down to join the palms again.

5. Coordinate your breathing with your arm movements. Keep your awareness on what you are doing as you practice.

6. Repeat five to ten times and rest.

Cautions and Comments:
- Breathe deeply and quietly through the nose during this whole exercise.
- Your movement should be graceful and constant. Always inhale lifting the arms and exhale lowering the arms.
- Children love this exercise!

Once you begin to practice breathing exercises, you may find that your nasal passages are blocked and need to be cleaned. The nasal wash cleansing technique can be most helpful, especially if you have a cold.

NASAL WASH

Benefits:
- Cleans, clears, and opens the nasal passages
- Removes wastes and toxins from the nasal passages
- Helps to prevent colds

Directions:
1. Fill a quart size watering can with body temperature water. Add a bit less than one teaspoon of sea salt to the water and mix well.

2. Lean over your sink as you place your right ear on your right hand and your elbow on the sink. Tilt your head so that your nasal passages are parallel to the sink.

3. Slowly begin to pour the water mixture into the top nostril and allow it to run out of the bottom nostril.

4. After half of the water is used, blow your nose on the clean side. Shift positions and wash the other nostril. Blow the other nostril.

Cautions and Comments:
- The salt-to-water ratio changes daily as your body chemistry changes. You may need to add a bit more than one teaspoon of salt some days, and a bit less on other days.

· If the water mixture burns you, you have used too little salt. If the mixture feels as if you are swimming under water, you have used too much salt. Adjust your cleansing mixture accordingly. The water should not pass into your throat, but only through your nasal passages. If you are getting water in your throat, adjust the position of your head so this does not happen.

Although suggested repetitions are indicated with each breathing exercise, if you like to do an exercise, do it as often as you like. By mastering the art of breathing during pregnancy, you will ensure relaxation between contractions during your labor, thereby helping to shorten your laboring time.

Three

Nutrition, Yoga, and Pregnancy

Look at the French word "la nourriture." Can you see a similarity to an English word? If you noticed the connection to the English verb "to nourish," you were right. "La nourriture" is the French word for food and it reflects a basic understanding of one of the most important values of eating. The food you eat should satisfy your tastes and desires while nourishing, developing, and sustaining both your body and your baby's body, brain, and being. During pregnancy you can begin to educate yourself about balanced eating in preparation for feeding your child in the coming years. In addition, by cultivating good nutritional habits, you can avoid many of the side effects of pregnancy. Recent research has indicated a definite link between proper nutrition, elimination of negative pregnancy experiences, and good health in the future baby. Only recently has it become clear that all things that are eaten can and do affect the growing baby. The varied and well balanced diet which is recommended within this chapter will be useful to you while you are expecting, while you are breastfeeding, and eventually for good health and vitality during your entire life. The diet is based on recommendations in the California Department of Health's report, *Nutrition During Pregnancy and Lactation* (1975), as well as on consultations with a clinical dietician.

THE YOGIC APPROACH TO FOOD

There are some simple yogic rules which should apply to your choice, preparation, and consumption of food:

1. Eat a large variety of foods from the four main food groups (proteins, calcium sources, whole grain and starchy products, and fresh fruits

and vegetables) which you try to balance. The variety of foods will provide all the essentials which your body needs to maintain itself and build a baby. The balance should increase your knowledge of nutrition as well as contributing to your good health.

2. Eat slowly and chew your food well. The digestion process begins in the mouth. Since stomach space becomes limited as the pregnancy progresses, you will ensure smoother digestion by chewing well.

3. Eat foods as close to their natural state as possible. Try to eat some raw foods daily. Foods in their natural state contain the energy of life (prana). Foods which are denatured by refining, preserving, canning, smoking, etc., lose this vital energy and are often "dead food." Choose fresh foods first, frozen foods second, and canned foods last.

4. When using processed foods, read the labels carefully to see what you and your baby are eating. (If you can't pronounce it, would you really want to eat it?) Many food additives have not been adequately tested, especially in relationship to cancer and birth defects. Why take chances? Additives to avoid are nitrites and nitrates; artificial colors and flavors; BHA and BHT; saccharin and cyclamates.

5. Cook your vegetables for a minimal time. Using a perforated steamer is best. You retain the most vitamins and minerals by quick cooking. When vegetables are cooked this way, they are brightly colored and extremely appealing to the eye. Use the water which is left in the bottom of the vegetable cooking pan as a highly nutritious low-calorie chilled drink or as a base for soups.

6. Eat five to six small meals a day. (Don't eat more, eat more often.) Eating smaller amounts will keep your energy levels stable. When you are feeling famished, you are more likely to reach for a candy bar than a salad. Eating small high-protein meals lessens the burden on your stomach and diminishes the likelihood of nausea and/or heartburn.

7. Eat only when your body feels hungry. Do not be pressured into eating when you are not really hungry. Do not feel that you need to conform to the usual standard times for meals. Learn to tune in to your body and detect when you are eating to fulfill hunger rather than eating to combat boredom or to be sociable.

8. Have a positive attitude toward the food you are eating. Close your eyes as you eat and really taste your food. Notice the texture of the food as well. Think of your food as the building blocks of your and your baby's health and development. Enjoy your food by really paying attention to how it tastes.

9. Do not eat when you are under emotional stress or are extremely tired. Wait until you have calmed down (do some "Rock-the-Baby"

breathing) or until after you have taken a nap. Your body may have difficulty digesting the food if you are in a heightened or depressed state. This is why indigestion usually goes with emotional upsets.

Following these simple and logical rules will help to improve your eating habits while ensuring more enjoyment from your meals.

HOW THE BODY WORKS

At one time or another during this pregnancy, you may have marveled at the workings of nature. Your baby began as two single cells and now may be kicking you as you read this. The workings of the body are truly miraculous and complicated. In order to maintain the body while building a baby inside, the proper "building materials" must be consumed each day.

Imagine that you are a worker within a vast factory and that you are trying to build a specific cell, say a baby heart cell. You have to gather all the basic ingredients from which a baby heart cell must be built. You discover a problem, one basic ingredient cannot be found. Your boss says to search all over to find the missing ingredient. You follow orders and look everywhere. You look in the body's stored reserves. You check into the areas where the body manufactures cells. But that special ingredient cannot be found today. "Well," says the boss, "I guess we can't do that job today. We'll have to wait until the missing ingredient comes in."

This is a very simplified imaginary story, but the main point is valid. If you are missing a basic ingredient, the cells in question cannot be manufactured. Although you may not want to know all about the inner workings of your body, it is extremely important to know which major ingredients have to be consumed each day to keep your body and your baby healthy.

Protein
Protein is used by the body to form the basic structure of every cell, as well as to build and maintain all the cells that compose the baby's body, the uterus, and the placenta. This nutrient plays a vital role in the production of brain cells in the growing fetus. Thus, adequate protein consumption is necessary for the future mental development of your child. Frequent high protein intake can eliminate the nausea of early pregnancy and prevent the toxemia which can develop in late pregnancy.

Many foods contain protein; however, there are complete and incomplete proteins. Women who are on vegetarian or other regulated diets while they are pregnant must be very careful to fulfill their daily complete protein requirement. It is possible to form complete proteins by mixing two incomplete proteins at the same meal. Reading and studying *Diet for a Small Planet* by Frances Moore Lappe (Ballantine Books, 1975), which contains thorough explanations of mixing incomplete proteins in the correct proportions to form complete proteins, should be mandatory for women on restricted diets. If you are on a limited diet, it is very important for you to keep a food diary (see instructions on page 36) so that you will be sure to eat adequate amounts of protein. Also vegetarian pregnant women should supplement their diet with B_{12} daily. Check with your doctor or midwife for amounts.

According to the Food and Nutrition Board of the National Academy of Sciences, the 1980 Recommended Daily Dietary Allowances (RDA) during pregnancy is a minimum of 74 grams of protein per day. Many nutritionists suggest 100 grams a day from the fifth month until the end of the pregnancy to insure adequate brain development in the child as well as good health in the mother. Study the illustrations of Group I Complete Protein Foods (Figures 3.2, 3.3, 3.4) for a more thorough understanding of complete and complementary protein foods and to know how much protein is in one serving of a food. A good pamphlet to read and study on prenatal nutrition is "As You Eat So Your Baby Grows" by Nikki Goldbeck, 1978. (See the Bibliography for mailing address.)

Calcium

This nutrient is the main ingredient for forming bones and teeth in your baby. Both calcium and phosphorous must be included in your daily food, especially during the last three months of your pregnancy when your baby's bones are developing. If your calcium intake is not high enough, your body will use its own bone cells to supply the baby. A lack of calcium in adequate supply within your diet can cause muscle cramps, (usually in the calves), sleeplessness, irritability, and increased tooth decay. Even if you do not like milk, you can fulfill your daily requirement by eating foods in Food Group II. Check Figure 3.5 on Calcium Sources for a better understanding of these foods. If you are not drinking milk or eating these other calcium food sources, you may want to talk to your doctor or midwife about supplementing your diet with calcium pills.

Vitamins

Vitamins are live substances within your food which play an important role in how well your body functions. Since they are live substances, they can be affected by heat, light, canning, freezing, and processing. That is why processed food products have to be vitamin-fortified. Fresh, raw foods contain high amounts of a wide variety of vitamins. However, if you allow your food to remain in the refrigerator for long periods of time, the vitamins deteriorate. The freezing and canning processes kill a high percentage of the vitamins in food. The vitamins found in oils such as Vitamins A, D, and E are fat soluble and can be stored in the body. An oversupply of these vitamins can be toxic and have very serious and dangerous effects on your body. That is why supplemental vitamins must be taken with care and knowledge. The water soluble vitamins such as the B complex (there are 11 recognized vitamins in this group) and C cannot be stored and must be replenished daily or symptoms of deficiency result. Vitamin C is very perishable and is destroyed by extreme heat and contact with the air. It is wise to prepare vitamin C rich foods right before you plan to eat them. If you are in a stressful situation, you will immediately burn the B and C vitamins present in your body. Smoking cigarettes severely depletes your vitamin C supply. If you continue to smoke while pregnant (although you really should not), you should increase your daily intake of Vitamin C by increasing the number of fruits and vegetables high in Vitamin C in your diet. The RDA for Vitamin C is 80 mgs. daily for pregnant women. For more details about vitamins and the foods in which they are found, see the Vitamin Chart (Figure 3.11) within this chapter.

Iron

Iron is an essential mineral which enables the hemoglobin (the red coloring matter in your blood) to carry oxygen to every cell of your body and the baby's. If your diet does not contain enough iron, you may develop anemia, fatigue, and shortness of breath. According to the Food and Nutrition Board of the National Academy of Sciences, the increased iron requirement cannot be met by the iron content of usual American diets or by the iron stores of many pregnant women. Therefore, an iron supplement of 30–60 mgs. daily should be taken. During the last three months of pregnancy, your baby's iron reserves are being formed; therefore, it is imperative to keep your iron intake high. The baby will be unable to utilize ingested iron very well in the first three months and so will use these reserves during that time.

Foods which are high in iron are fresh fruits (especially apricots), green leafy vegetables, prune juice, almonds, liver, egg yolk, wheat germ, and blackstrap molasses. You may want to try Aunt Mollie's Famous Chopped Liver Spread (Figure 3.14), which has been included in this chapter. It contains very high iron levels and makes a tasty sandwich spread.

If you are a vegetarian or do not care for liver, you may want to add one tablespoon of blackstrap molasses (3.2 mgs. of iron) to each glass of milk that you drink. You can also add blackstrap molasses to the Fruity Milkshake Recipe (Figure 3.15) contained within this chapter.

Almost all pregnant women take an iron supplement of 30–60 mgs. in pill form. You should be aware that there are a variety of supplements available. Often pregnant women find that they become very constipated from these supplements. Ferrous sulfate should not be taken during pregnancy because it destroys Vitamin E very quickly. Other kinds of iron supplements which have been found to be effective but not constipating are ferrous gluconate, ferrous fumurate (FemIron) or ferrous sulfate with molybdenum (Mol-Iron). Iron supplementation should be continued all during the time you breastfeed or bottle-feed your baby.

Weight Gain

Most pregnant women are very concerned about the amount of weight they gain during the waiting months. A weight gain is a natural indicator that the body is changing and growing to facilitate the development of the baby. The dietary requirements which have been recommended in this chapter are necessary to accommodate the increase in your body's metabolism and tissue production as well as the growth of the baby. Weight gain during pregnancy should, therefore, be regarded as a positive aspect of the pregnancy. Your mental attitude about this change in your body shape will have a very definite effect on you, so you should spend some time sorting out your feelings.

Most doctors and midwives agree that a weight gain of 21–30 pounds is desirable for a healthy baby. During your prenatal checkups, you will be monitored very carefully for there should be a definite pattern to this weight gain. During the first trimester there should be a very minimal weight gain of two to four lbs. During the second trimester, when much growth takes place, you should gain about three to four lbs. a month. During the last trimester your weight gain will reflect the baby putting on weight in preparation for birth. You should not limit your diet, especially during the last trimester, for it will directly deprive your baby of good birth weight and a chance for good health.

Vegetarian Diets and Pregnancy

Yoga and vegetarian eating seem to be naturally linked in this country. However, to thrive on a vegetarian diet, you must have a basic knowledge of nutrition and complementary proteins. This takes some study and understanding. Often people become vegetarians without this prior knowledge with very disastrous results, such as lack of energy, irritability, and illness.

You should not consider becoming a vegetarian when you are pregnant because the bodily needs for complete protein are very high. It would be very difficult to completely fulfill these needs without some prior experience working with complementary proteins and unfamiliar foods. You can, however, try introducing more high-protein vegetarian meals into your diet to see how you react. (Check the Bibliography for suggested cookbooks.)

HERBS AND PREGNANCY

The use of natural remedies has been growing in popularity during the past few years. Many people are turning to herbal remedies because they prefer a more natural approach. With the relationship between increased stress and caffeine consumption being more clearly understood and accepted, more people are turning to caffeine-free herbal teas. Much knowledge concerning herbs and herbal cures is being published and read at the present time. From a yogic point of view, herbal teas can be most beneficial if you learn some basic information about the herbs that you are drinking. You must remember that herbs are a form of medicine and that some herbs can have a very negative effect on your body.

Herb tea can be prepared in an enamel pan or in a cup. To prepare one cup, pour boiling water on one teaspoon of the dried plant or tea bag and let it steep for five to ten minutes. It will not usually get as dark as English, Indian, or Chinese tea. If using loose herbs, strain and drink while still warm; add some honey for sweetness or a squeeze of lemon.

Historically, Red Raspberry leaf tea Rubus Ideaus (Figure 3.1) has been noted as the best and most helpful herbal tea for pregnancy, birth, and lactation. Red Raspberry leaves have a very beneficial effect on the female reproductive organs. Many women who have consumed this tea during labor and after the baby's birth report an easier and less painful birthing process and a reduction in afterbirth cramps. This tea has been quite effectively used to minimize menstrual cramps as well. It has a mild flavor and is available at most health food stores for a nominal cost. It can be drunk three to four times a day all during pregnancy to increase the strength and viability of the uterus and to prepare the body for birth. Red Raspberry leaf is also available from the Celestial Seasoning Herb Tea Co. under the name "Winterberry." As Winterberry tea, it is mixed with some mint tea for added flavor. It is very nice hot or iced. Herb teas are now being sold at supermarkets, so check the herb tea shelf for a new taste treat.

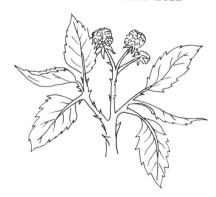

Figure 3.1 Red Rasberry Leaf (Rubus Ideaus).

Herbal Teas for Other Uses

Nausea

Peppermint tea (Mentha piperita) is helpful for eliminating nausea or upset stomach. Warm tea is often more helpful than cold. (Figure 3.2) *Camomile* tea (Matricaria or anthemis nobilis) relieves many ailments, especially those in the womb and the stomach. It helps to eliminate vomiting if consumed in the morning . It has been known to relieve intestinal gas as well.

Sleeplessness

Camomile is very soothing when drunk while still hot with a bit of honey if you prefer. Celestial Seasoning Herb Tea Co. produces a mixture called "Sleepytime," which contains camomile and other assorted herbs. This is a very soothing, and often sleep-inducing, safe tea for pregnancy (Figure 3.3).

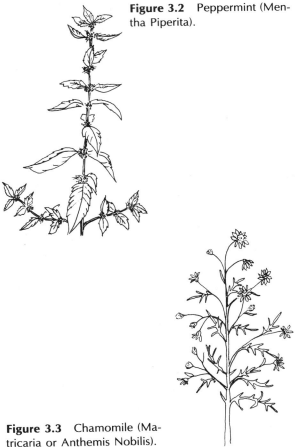

Figure 3.2 Peppermint (Mentha Piperita).

Figure 3.3 Chamomile (Matricaria or Anthemis Nobilis).

Birthing

Red Raspberry (Rubus Ideaus)—As already mentioned, this plant is known to promote a relaxed delivery and is an astringent.

Spikenard tea (Aralia racemosa) is known as a blood purifier and is recommended during the last six weeks of pregnancy in combination with Red Raspberry leaf.

Postpartum Healing

Comfrey tea (Symphytum officinale) is exceedingly helpful for healing wounds. Crushing a fresh leaf to release the juices and placing it over your sanitary pad will help to heal up the episiotomy or other tears. If you prefer, you can make a tea from three teaspoons of comfrey leaf and one cup of hot water, simmered for 20 minutes. After straining and cooling the tea, a soft cloth can be dipped into the warm tea and be applied to the wound area to promote healing (Figure 3.4).

Cracked Nipples

Aloe Vera (Aloe Vera) is good for cracked nipples. Cut a piece of the Aloe Vera plant and apply the moist part to the damaged nipple. Repeat a few minutes later after the nipple has dried. At the next feeding use the other breast only. Before you use the treated nipple, wash it carefully with warm water. Repeat the Aloe Vera application after each feeding until the nipple has healed (Figure 3.5).

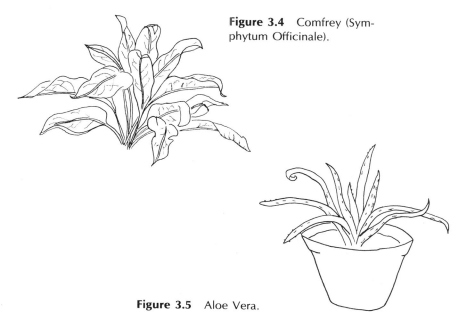

Figure 3.4 Comfrey (Symphytum Officinale).

Figure 3.5 Aloe Vera.

Herbs Which Can Be Dangerous

Before using any substance, you should be aware of its effects on your body. The following herbs can have very negative effects if used in the wrong proportion or at the wrong time. If you are not working with a trained herbologist, you should avoid the following substances during pregnancy and lactation:

Lobelia (Lobelia inflata) is a very strong herb which can act as a stimulant and as a relaxant. Excessive dosages can induce continual vomiting. *Peach tree leaves* must be used in specific quantities because the leaves and flowers contain small amounts of hydrocyanic acid, which is poisonous. Excess use of these leaves can cause diarrhea. *Blue Cohosh* is often irritating to the mucous membranes, but it has been used by women to strengthen their uterine contractions during labor. Other herbal teas to avoid are *Golden Seal, Yarrow, Valerian, Tansy, Cotton Root, Motherwort, Couchgrass, Rue, Pennyroyal, Vervain* and *St. John's Wort.* These teas can cause the uterus to begin contracting and thus cause a miscarriage.

You may want to check the bibliography for a listing of books on herbs so that you can become more familiar with their properties and benefits. Always check the ingredient lists when buying herbal teas to see that they do not contain the above-mentioned detrimental herbs. New herbal teas which are "pregnancy brews" are available at some health food stores. If you buy a "pregnancy tea," it should contain Red Raspberry leaf in combination with two or three other herbs. Experimenting with the different tastes which herbal teas can provide can be a new and interesting aspect of your pregnancy.

CAUTIONS AND COMMENTS FOR PREGNANCY NUTRITION

- Do not take any drugs (over-the-counter included) unless specifically recommended by your doctor or midwife. This includes marijuana, LSD, etc.

- Do not take diuretics, (water pills) which can flush important minerals out of your system.

- Minimize your consumption of caffeine foods such as coffee, leaf tea, cola drinks, and cocoa. The connection between high caffeine intake and birth defects is now being researched. Substitute herbal teas, grain coffee substitutes like Postum and Pero, unsweetened fruit juices, mineral water or iced water with half of a fresh lemon squeezed into it.

- Do not diet during pregnancy even if you were overweight when you became pregnant. You may cause birth defects in your future child.

- Either do not smoke or cut down to as few cigarettes daily as you can. The smoke in your system deprives your unborn child of necessary oxygen. Low birth weight or premature babies are often born to mothers who smoke. Smoking pregnant women should increase their Vitamin C intake.

- Do not take mind-altering drugs such as LSD or marijuana, for research is not complete on the effect of these drugs on the unborn child.

- Alcohol, consumed in even moderate amounts, may cause birth defects in your child in the form of both physical and behavioral abnormalities. You should consume no more than two mixed drinks (containing a total of 3 ounces of hard liquor) or two glasses of beer or wine each day. Drink mineral water with half of a lime squeezed in and make believe it's a Gin and Tonic. Create your own non-alcoholic drinks.

- Try to keep your intake of chemical additives to a minimum. Luncheon meats contain nitrates and nitrites. Substitute sliced home cooked turkey, chicken, chopped liver or roast beef.

- Do not fast during pregnancy. Going without food for even 24 hours is not good for your growing baby.

- Drink six to eight glasses of liquid daily in the form of water, unsweetened fruit juices, herbal teas, grain coffee substitutes, vegetable juices, etc.

- Salt your food to taste. If swelling occurs in your legs, you should talk to your doctor or midwife. Do not eliminate salt from your diet, for it is necessary for your body's metabolism.

- Snack often during the day choosing foods that are nutritious and also tasty. See the suggested snack recipes which are illustrated within this chapter (Figures 3.12, 3.14, 3.15).

- Try to keep your white sugar consumption to a minimum. Use honey or molasses instead, but sparingly. Sugar contributes to increased tooth decay as well as to emotional ups and downs.

- Keep a food diary for several days each month so that you will be able to check that you are eating foods from the four basic food groups. Using a food diary is an easy way to learn all the fundamentals of good nutrition.

- Avoid greasy fried foods, sweets, fats, rich pastries, fat drippings, and gravies.

Most important of all things that contribute to a happy and healthy pregnancy is a positive mental attitude. Try to keep in positive spaces as you eat, nourish, and build your baby.

CHECKLIST FOR DAILY FOOD DIARY
DURING PREGNANCY

Remember to eat the correct amount daily from each food group. Check illustrations in this chapter for detailed food group listings and caloric values.

Servings Per Day:

Group I	Complete protein Meat (Figure 3.2) Meatless (Figure 3.3) Complementary (Figure 3.4)	Six to eight 1-oz. servings
Group II	Calcium sources (Figure 3.5)	Four servings (1 serving = 8 oz. of milk or the equivalent)
Group III	Whole grain products (Figure 3.13) and starchy vegetables (Figure 3.6)	Four servings (1 serving = 1 slice of bread or its equivalent)
Group IV	Fruits and vegetables with Vitamin C (Figure 3.7)	One serving (1 serving = 1 orange or its equivalent)
	Leafy green vegetables with Vitamin A, folic acid and iron (Figure 3.8)	Two servings (1 serving = 1 cup or its equivalent)
	Other fruits and vegetables with Vitamin A (Figure 3.9)	One serving (½ cup or its equivalent)
Others	Butter; vegetable oil; fortified margarine; salt to taste	One to two tablespoons
	Liquids	Six to eight glasses a day
	Snacks (Dried fruits, unsalted nuts, sunflower seeds, unsalted popcorn, or see Suggested Snacks, Figures 3.12, 15, 16)	One to three daily

FOOD DIARY

Use a food diary as your guide for evaluating your diet. Write down in a notebook or on a sheet of paper what you eat throughout the day. Include breakfast, lunch, and supper, as well as mid-morning, afternoon, and evening snacks. Does your daily diet contain the prescribed number of servings from each food group? Is it varied? Are you eating four to six small meals a day? Are you eating only when hungry?

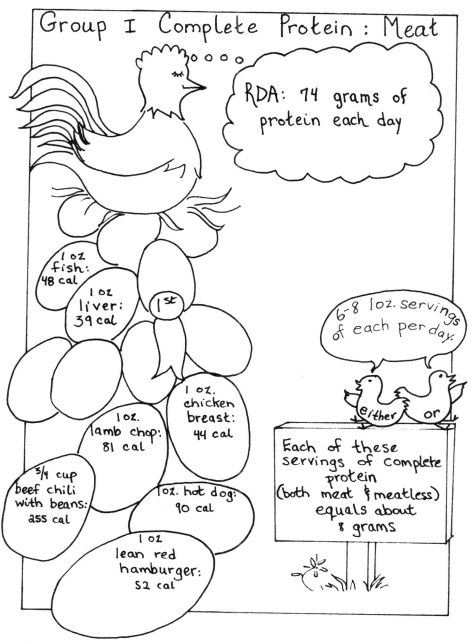

Figure 3.6

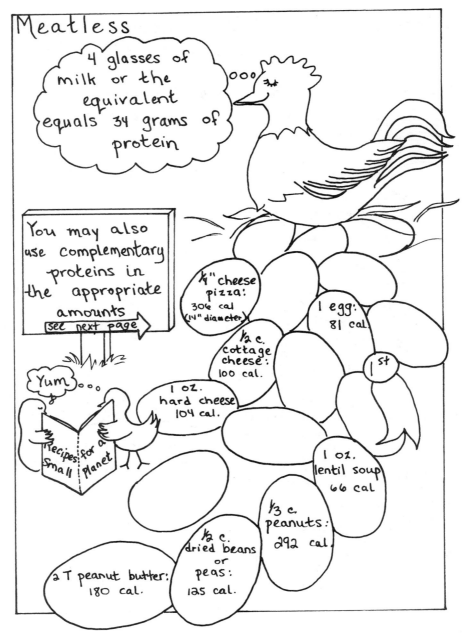

Figure 3.7

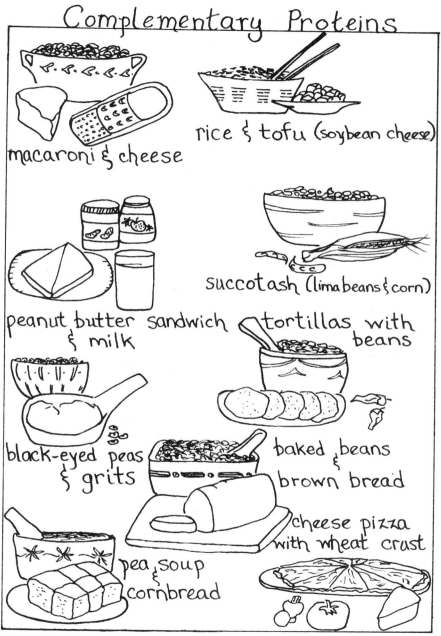

Complementary Proteins

macaroni & cheese

rice & tofu (soybean cheese)

peanut butter sandwich & milk

succotash (lima beans & corn)

black-eyed peas & grits

tortillas with beans

baked beans & brown bread

pea soup & cornbread

cheese pizza with wheat crust

Figure 3.8

Figure 3.9

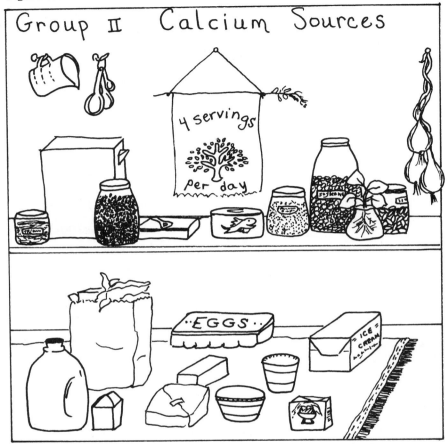

Group Ⅱ Calcium Sources

4 servings per day

⅓ c. dry milk powder: 72 cal.
2½ oz. sardines: 138
½ c. salmon with bones: 173
3 T sesame seeds: 105
2⅘ c. soybeans: 283
2 6 oz. cakes of tofu: 144
1 c. milk - whole: 161, skim: 88
1½ c. ice cream: 450

1 c. almonds: 872
1 c. baked custard: 305
1 c. chocolate pudding: 382
1⅓ oz. cheese: 160
8 oz. turnip greens or kale: 73
8 oz. plain yogurt: 125
1⅓ c. cottage cheese: 280
1 c. buttermilk: 88

Group III Whole Grain Products and Starchy Vegetables

minimum of 4 servings per day

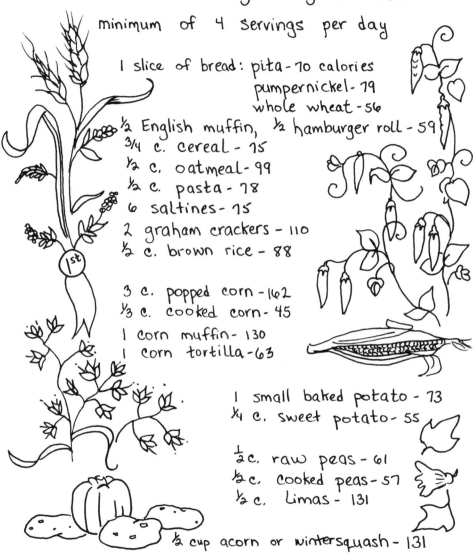

1 slice of bread: pita - 70 calories
                   pumpernickel - 79
                   whole wheat - 56

½ English muffin, ½ hamburger roll - 59
¾ c. cereal - 75
½ c. oatmeal - 99
½ c. pasta - 78
6 saltines - 75
2 graham crackers - 110
½ c. brown rice - 88

3 c. popped corn - 162
⅓ c. cooked corn - 45
1 corn muffin - 130
1 corn tortilla - 63

1 small baked potato - 73
¼ c. sweet potato - 55

½ c. raw peas - 61
½ c. cooked peas - 57
½ c. Limas - 131

½ cup acorn or wintersquash - 131

Figure 3.10

41

Figure 3.11

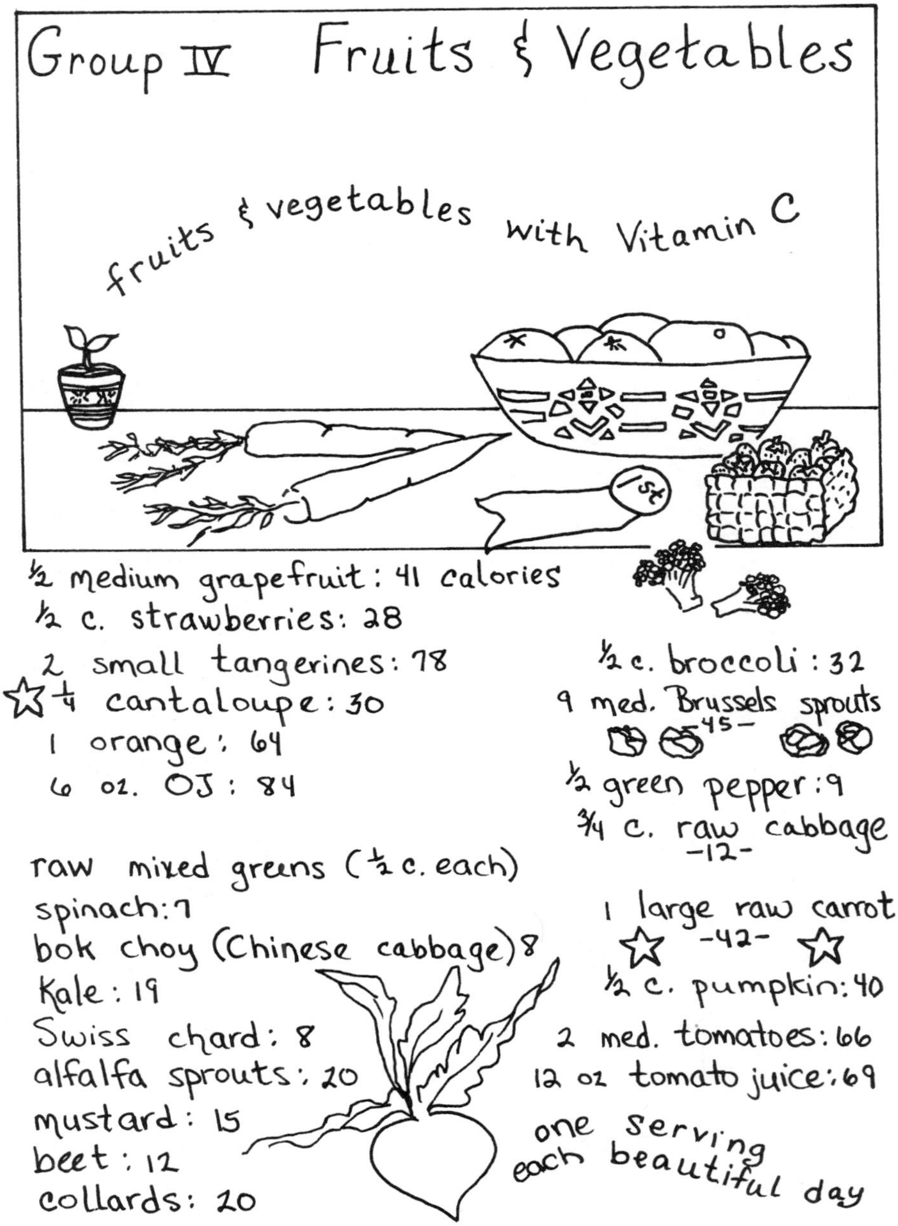

Group IV   Fruits & Vegetables

fruits & vegetables with Vitamin C

½ medium grapefruit: 41 calories
½ c. strawberries: 28
2 small tangerines: 78
☆ ¼ cantaloupe: 30
1 orange: 64
6 oz. OJ: 84

½ c. broccoli: 32
9 med. Brussels sprouts
  -45-
½ green pepper: 9
¾ c. raw cabbage
  -12-

1 large raw carrot
☆ -42- ☆
½ c. pumpkin: 40

2 med. tomatoes: 66
12 oz tomato juice: 69

raw mixed greens (½ c. each)
spinach: 7
bok choy (Chinese cabbage) 8
kale: 19
Swiss chard: 8
alfalfa sprouts: 20
mustard: 15
beet: 12
collards: 20

one serving
each beautiful day

More Group IV Fruits & Veggies

Leafy, green vegetables ⓦ Vit. A, Folic Acid, & Iron

1 c. asparagus: 35 calories
1 c. broccoli (cooked): 40
9 med. Brussels sprouts: 45
1 c. cabbage: 16
1 c. { romaine
       endive   } 10
       escarole }

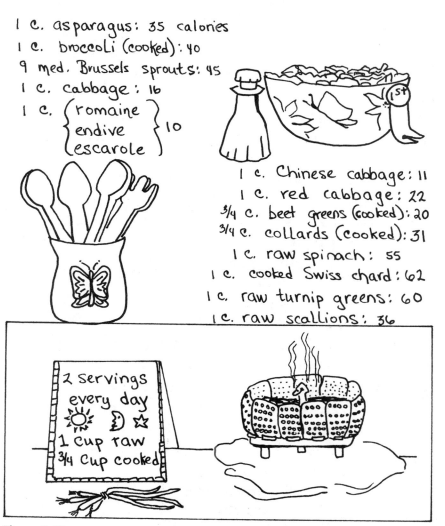

1 c. Chinese cabbage: 11
1 c. red cabbage: 22
3/4 c. beet greens (cooked): 20
3/4 c. collards (cooked): 31
1 c. raw spinach: 55
1 c. cooked Swiss chard: 62
1 c. raw turnip greens: 60
1 c. raw scallions: 36

2 servings every day ☀ ☽ ☆
1 cup raw
3/4 cup cooked

Figure 3.12

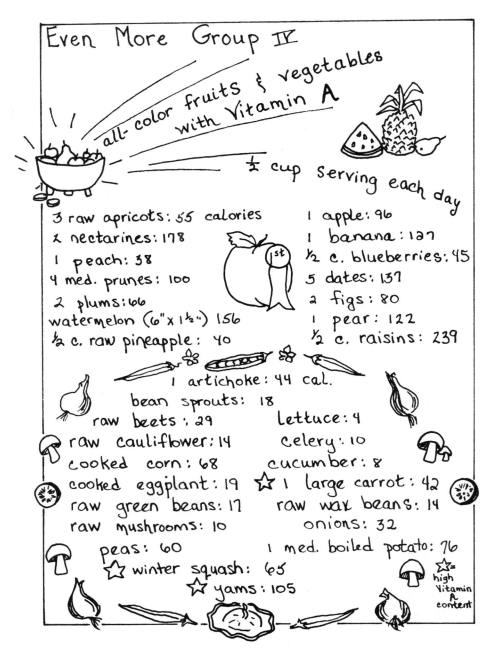

Even More Group IV

all-color fruits & vegetables with Vitamin A

½ cup serving each day

3 raw apricots: 55 calories
2 nectarines: 178
1 peach: 38
4 med. prunes: 100
2 plums: 66
watermelon (6"x 1½") 156
½ c. raw pineapple: 40

1 apple: 96
1 banana: 127
½ c. blueberries: 45
5 dates: 137
2 figs: 80
1 pear: 122
½ c. raisins: 239

1 artichoke: 44 cal.
bean sprouts: 18
raw beets: 29
raw cauliflower: 14
cooked corn: 68
cooked eggplant: 19
raw green beans: 17
raw mushrooms: 10
peas: 60
☆ winter squash: 65
☆ yams: 105

lettuce: 4
celery: 10
cucumber: 8
☆ 1 large carrot: 42
raw wax beans: 14
onions: 32
1 med. boiled potato: 76

☆= high Vitamin A content

Figure 3.13

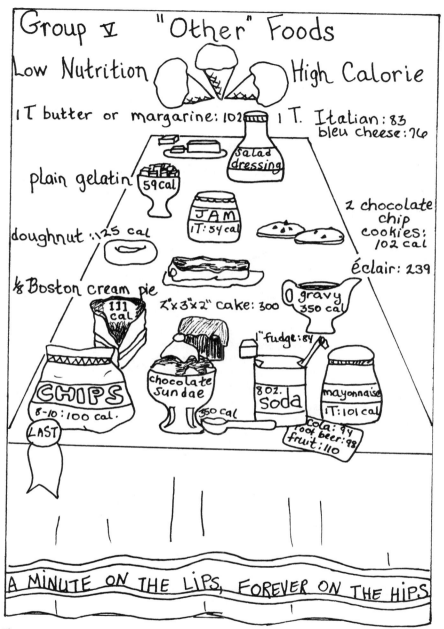

Figure 3.14

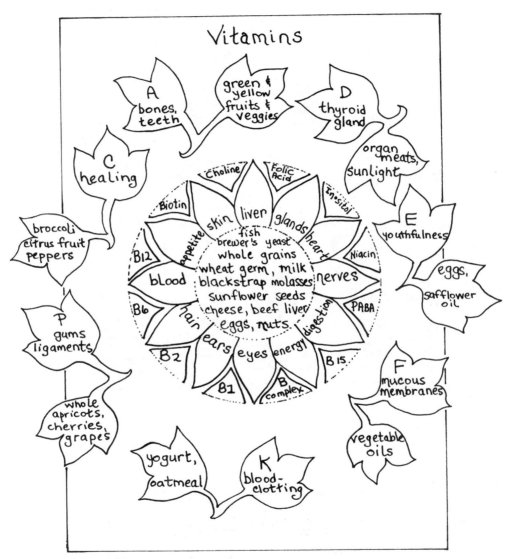

Figure 3.15

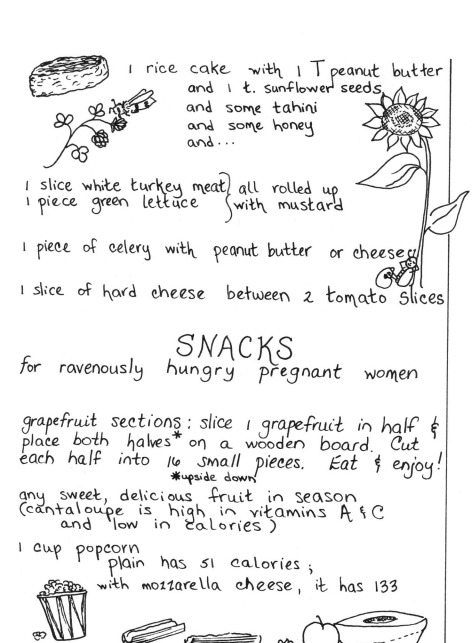

1 rice cake with 1 T peanut butter
and 1 t. sunflower seeds
and some tahini
and some honey
and...

1 slice white turkey meat⎫ all rolled up
1 piece green lettuce   ⎬ with mustard

1 piece of celery with peanut butter or cheese

1 slice of hard cheese between 2 tomato slices

SNACKS
for ravenously hungry pregnant women

grapefruit sections: slice 1 grapefruit in half &
place both halves* on a wooden board. Cut
each half into 16 small pieces. Eat & enjoy!
            *upside down

any sweet, delicious fruit in season
(cantaloupe is high in vitamins A & C
    and low in calories)

1 cup popcorn
        plain has 51 calories;
        with mozzarella cheese, it has 133

Figure 3.16

47

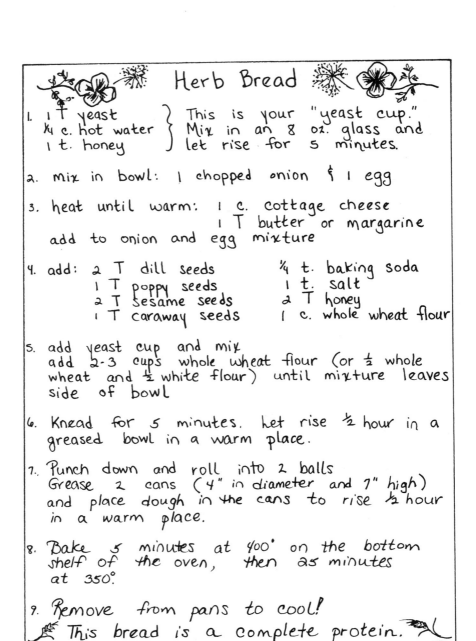

Herb Bread

1. 1 T yeast
   1/4 c. hot water   } This is your "yeast cup."
   1 t. honey   Mix in an 8 oz. glass and
                            let rise for 5 minutes.

2. mix in bowl: 1 chopped onion & 1 egg

3. heat until warm: 1 c. cottage cheese
                    1 T butter or margarine
   add to onion and egg mixture

4. add: 2 T dill seeds   1/4 t. baking soda
        1 T poppy seeds   1 t. salt
        2 T sesame seeds   2 T honey
        1 T caraway seeds   1 c. whole wheat flour

5. add yeast cup and mix
   add 2-3 cups whole wheat flour (or 1/2 whole
   wheat and 1/2 white flour) until mixture leaves
   side of bowl

6. Knead for 5 minutes. Let rise 1/2 hour in a
   greased bowl in a warm place.

7. Punch down and roll into 2 balls
   Grease 2 cans (4" in diameter and 7" high)
   and place dough in the cans to rise 1/2 hour
   in a warm place.

8. Bake 5 minutes at 400° on the bottom
   shelf of the oven, then 25 minutes
   at 350°.

9. Remove from pans to cool!
   This bread is a complete protein.

Figure 3.17

48

Aunt Mollie's Famous Chopped Liver

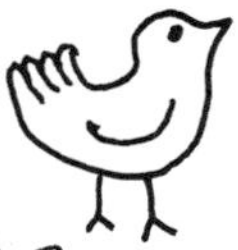

1 lb. chicken livers
2 large onions, chopped
3-4 T. vegetable oil
4 eggs, hard-boiled
¼ t. salt
pepper to taste
½ T mayonnaise

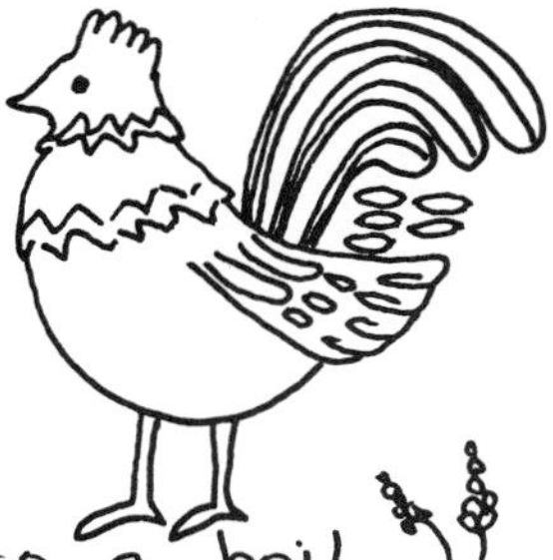

1. Bring a large pan of water to a boil. Add chicken livers and boil 8-10 minutes. (Do not overcook. Check for doneness by removing one liver and slicing it. If tan, not red, inside- it is done.)

2. While liver is boiling, sauté onion in oil until the onion is translucent. Boil eggs at the same time.

3. Strain livers to remove excess water. Place livers, onions and the oil they were cooked in, peeled boiled eggs, and salt in food processor. Process 20-30 seconds. If you prefer a smooth spread, process longer. If you do not have a food processor, chop in wooden bowl to desired consistency. Add mayonnaise if you like.

Note: If liver is overcooked, add 1-2 T of water. Do not add extra oil. Adjust seasoning to your taste. You can decrease eggs or onions or add more spices.

☆ This makes an excellent hor d'oeuvre spread and is great on sandwiches. It is a most palatable way to eat liver and keep your iron up.

Figure 3.18

Peanut Butter Candy:
½ c. natural peanut butter
¼ c. powdered milk
⅓ c. honey (or less)
⅓ c. carob powder
(optional)

Mix ingredients well.
Shape into small balls
and roll in shredded
coconut and/or sesame
seeds. Place in small
pieces of waxed paper.
Keep refrigerated in
warm weather.

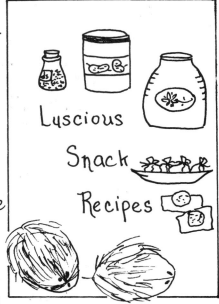

Luscious

Snack

Recipes

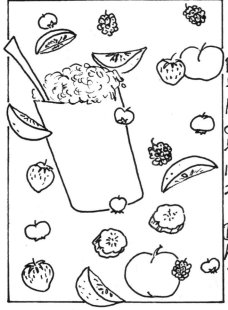

Fruity Milkshake:
(120-150 calories)

Pour ½ glass of milk into
food processor or blender.
Add 2 ice cubes and 2
of any of the following:
½ banana / 10 strawberries
10 raspberries / ½ peach
20 blueberries / ½ orange
        ½ nectarine
Blend 1-2 minutes. Add
honey if you like.
Drink it before the
        foam disappears!

Figure 3.19

Tofu Spread:

10 oz. tofu (bean curd)
½ c. natural peanut butter
2 T. lemon juice
2 T. honey

Blend or mix in
food processor.
Refrigerate in a
covered jar.

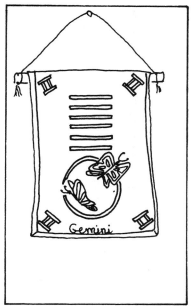

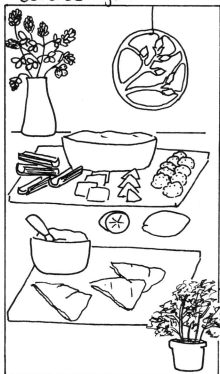

Figure 3.20

Humus Spread or Dip
(a complete protein)

½ c. chick peas (cooked or canned)
1-2 cloves minced garlic
½ t. salt, dash of tamari
juice of 1 medium lemon
½ c. tahini 2 tblsp. sesame seeds
¼ c. chopped parsley
¼ c. minced scallions
black pepper & cayenne
Whirl in food processor
for 1 minute. Or chop
in blender & mix in a
separate bowl.

Four

Natural Aids for Some Common Pregnancy Complaints

The experience of pregnancy is as varied as the babies that arrive when the pregnancy culminates. The variety of pregnancy complaints covers a wide scope. Some of these complaints are very subtle and disappear very quickly while others may linger for months and sometimes last during the entire pregnancy. Since medication of any sort is usually forbidden during pregnancy, natural remedies which can eliminate or minimize the problem are most useful.

This chapter will discuss some of pregnancy's most common complaints and some natural remedies using yoga physical postures, dietary changes, yogic breathing, cleansing and relaxing techniques as well as general information to relieve a worried mind. I have indicated on which page you can find the appropriate asana described in complete detail. It is very important to stress that any dietary supplement such as vitamins must be approved by your doctor or midwife. Do not take any pills without your doctor's or midwife's consent.

Although all the information which is contained in this chapter is accurate and useful, your situation may be different from the general situation which has been described. Dosages of vitamins vary according to your specific situation. After you have obtained your doctor's or midwife's approval for using the exercises and dietary changes, keep them well informed about your progress in alleviating the complaint. You will notice that many of the most common pregnancy complaints are due to inadequate or improperly balanced nutritional patterns. By keeping track of what you are eating via a food diary, you will be sure to know that your diet is nutritionally sufficient for both you and the baby.

Backache

Useful Asanas:
1. Good posture (p. 121)
2. Alternate Leg Stretch to the side (p. 124)
3. Bridge (pp. 86–88)
4. Lower Back Rocker (p. 88)
5. Pelvic Rocking (pp. 86–88)
6. Pendulum Legs (pp. 114–16)
7. Spinal Twist (pp. 85–86)
8. Salute to the Child (pp. 96–109)
9. Universal Pose (pp. 116–17)
10. Hip Rotater: stand with your feet two feet apart. Begin to move your hips in a circle while you keep your shoulders still. Circle five times in both directions. Do this while you are preparing breakfast to get your lower back loose and pain free.

Cautions:
1. Do not do forward bending, lying on tummy, strong upward stretching exercises.
2. Do not wear high heeled shoes. They increase the likelihood of backache.

Tips and Information:
1. Practice the "Basic Nine" daily to eliminate backache.
2. Learn to take two to three minute stretch periods during the day.
3. Do not stay in one position for long periods of time.

Constipation

Useful Asanas:
Knee to Chest Position (on side):

Lie on your side. Bend top knee and place it near your chest.

Wrap your arm around your knee and hold, breathing normally for 15–20 seconds.

Keep head on mat throughout. Repeat on other side.

Repeat two to five times.

Dietary Changes:
1. Add fresh and dried fruits (prunes, raisins, figs, etc.) to daily diet.

2. Eat fresh vegetables and salads containing a variety of raw green and colored vegetables daily.

3. Drink six to eight glasses of liquid (some water) each day.

4. Eat whole grain breads, cereals, and whole bran flakes. Begin with two teaspoons in a glass of apple juice twice a day. The bran may cause some gas until your system gets used to it.

Breathing and Relaxation Exercises:
"Rock-the-Baby" breath will stimulate the intestinal area. Do ten breaths (pp. 14–16).

Cautions:
Do not take bottled laxatives without your doctor's or midwife's approval.

Tips and Information:
1. Increasing progesterone in your system makes bowels less efficient.

2. Walking a mile a day is very helpful.

3. Set a regular time each day to move your bowels.

4. Keeping your feet and legs elevated on a footstool during elimination helps to move the bowels by releasing the anal muscles.

5. An enema using body temperature water may be used occasionally if all else fails.

Gas (Flatulence)

Useful Asanas:
1. Zen Sitting Position for five minutes after meals helps digestion (p. 93)

2. Squatting postures, if you do not have varicose veins (p. 15)

3. Knees on Chest and Rock (if comfortable) (p. 88)

4. Knee to Chest (on side) (p. 54)

Dietary Changes:
1. Eat four to five small meals a day.

2. Chew your food slowly and well.

3. Avoid foods which cause you to have gas. Keep a food diary to obtain this information.

4. Cook your foods quickly using a perforated steamer instead of boiling for long periods of time.

5. To reduce gas-causing sulphur compounds in beans (including pinto, garbanzo, navy, etc.), bring one cup of beans to a boil in five cups of water. Boil one minute. Drain and add five fresh cups of water. Bring to second boil and cook as per directions.

Cautions:
Gas may be due to eating foods together which cause gas to develop in your body. Keep a food diary to check your food combinations.

Tips and Information:
1. Walking one mile a day should help digestion and elimination.
2. Setting a regular time to move your bowels will be helpful as well.

Groin spasm, stitch, or pressure

Useful Asanas:
1. Half Bow on Side (p. 90)
2. Half Bow standing (p. 113)
3. Salute to the Child, #7 and #8 (pp. 103–6)
4. Squatting positions
5. Knee to Chest (on side) (p. 54)
6. Pregnancy Triangle (pp. 109–11). Do this with both legs straight.
7. Alternate Leg Stretch to the Side (p. 124)

Breathing and Relaxation Exercises:
1. Deep breathe when spasm is occurring (pp. 13–14).
2. Relax in a left side lying position until spasm is over (pp. 153–54).

Tips and Information:
1. Often this is felt as a stitch on the right side. The round ligaments connecting the corners of the uterus to the pubic area will kink and go into a spasm.
2. In the later months, lower groin pressure may develop. Exercising daily can help to alleviate this condition.

Headaches

Useful Asanas:
1. Neck Rolls in a cross-legged or zen sitting position (pp. 79–81)
2. Self-massage of neck and face (pp. 181–82)
3. Partner massage (pp. 177–80)

Dietary Changes:

1. Drink strong peppermint, rosemary, catnip, or sage tea and lie down for 20 minutes for Complete Relaxation.

2. Avoid foods with MSG (monosodium glutamate) (often in Chinese food) and nitrates (in luncheon meat.) Both these substances can cause headaches in sensitive people.

3. Avoid alcoholic beverages including wine and champagne.

4. For sinus headaches, cut down on dairy products in your diet. Increase intake of citrus fruits and fresh leafy vegetables.

Breathing and Relaxation Exercises:

1. Alternate Nostril Breathing. Do ten rounds in cross–legged position. *Do not do this lying down!* (pp. 16–18)

2. Complete Relaxation for 10 to 20 minutes (p. 96)

3. Baby Meditation

Cautions:

1. Consult your doctor or midwife immediately for severe or long–lasting headaches.

2. Do not sleep with your head under the covers for this creates a shortage of oxygen and then a headache.

3. Minimize coffee consumption; it often causes headaches in pregnant women.

4. Dairy products can cause extra mucous, sinus problems, and often headaches.

Tips and Information:

1. Walk one mile a day while practicing deep breathing.

2. Make "Rock-the-Baby" breath part of your daily routine.

3. Press hot wet towels on your head and face under a hot shower for sinus headaches.

4. Lightly massage sinus areas on forehead and cheeks to stimulate drainage of sinuses.

Heartburn

Useful Asanas:

1. Salute to the Child (pp. 96–109)

2. Spinal Twist (pp. 85–86)

Dietary Changes:
1. Eat four to six small meals a day.
2. Drink one tablespoon of cream, milk, or buttermilk before eating to coat and soothe stomach.

Breathing and Relaxation Exercises:
1. "Rock-the-Baby" breath (pp. 13–14)
2. Baby breath (pp. 14–16)

Cautions:
1. Do not take baking soda or Alka Seltzer. Both have a very high salt content which may cause water retention and swelling.
2. Use alcohol and coffee in moderation for both have been found to contribute to heartburn in pregnant women.
3. *Do not eat highly spiced or greasy foods.*

Tips and Information:
1. The burning sensation results from stomach fluids re–entering the esophagus (food tube) because of the size of the uterus.
2. Gelusil, Milk of Magnesia tablets, or Maalox are often recommended but *check with your doctor or midwife before taking an antacid.*
3. Keep moving if heartburn strikes and do some "Rock-the-Baby" breathing.
4. Have faith! It ends with the birth of the baby.

Hemorrhoids

Useful Asanas:
1. Anal Lock (in Basic Nine) (pp. 92–94)
2. Pelvic Floor Exercises (pp. 129–31)
3. Cross-legged Sitting Position and Rocking (pp. 122–23)
4. Fish Position (pp. 117–19)
5. Salute to the Child (Try rocking side to side in position #5)

Dietary Changes:
1. Increase roughage in your diet to soften stools and make elimination easier. Foods which increase roughage are: raw vegetables, fruits, dried fruits, whole bran flakes, whole grain breads.
2. Drink six to eight glasses of liquid a day such as water, juices, herbal teas and milk.

Breathing and Relaxation Exercises:

1. Coordinate breathing as you practice the Anal Lock: exhale–lock, inhale–release (pp. 92–94)

2. While you are moving your bowels, do not hold your breath. Instead, inhale and exhale continually.

Cautions:

1. Hard stools may be quite painful and cause bleeding.

2. Do not stay on the toilet bowl too long. Eliminate and leave. Make your living room your reading room, not the bathroom.

Tips and Information:

1. Practice the Anal Lock in the shower. (Fold a washcloth until it is 4" by 1". Wet the cloth and wring it out. Place the washcloth on the hemorrhoidal area and practice the Anal Lock. You should be able to hold the washcloth there. Relax the muscles and let the washcloth drop. Repeat five to ten times.)

2. Keep your feet and legs elevated on a high footstool while eliminating. This helps to move the bowels by releasing the anal muscles.

3. Use cold compresses with witch hazel.

4. Walking one mile a day helps digestion and elimination.

5. Keep the bowel area clean by washing completely with warm water after each bowel movement. Then apply oil or A&D ointment.

6. Soak in a warm, cold, or tepid bathtub.

Insomnia

Useful Asanas and Cleansing Techniques:

1. Salute to the Child, two to five repetitions (pp. 96–109)

2. A hot bath right before bed can help to make you drowsy.

Dietary Changes:

1. Drink hot milk with powdered milk, honey, or molasses half hour before you go to bed.

2. Herb teas such as camomile, marjoram, and lemon balm are known for their sleep producing qualities. Try a hot cup of tea with honey or lemon before bed or in the middle of the night.

3. A B-vitamin deficiency in your diet often can cause insomnia. Increase your intake of foods rich in Vitamin B. Keeping a food diary can help diagnose this situation.

Breathing and Relaxation Exercises:

1. Anti-Insomnia Breath (pp. 18–19)

2. Have your mate give you a soothing massage.

Cautions:

1. *Do not take any sleeping pills when you are pregnant.*

2. Do not force yourself to sleep if you are really not tired. Read or do quiet chores until you feel sleepy.

Tips and Information:

1. Insomnia is very common during the last weeks of pregnancy when finding a comfortable sleeping position is difficult.

2. This is the natural way to prepare for the 3:00 A.M. feeding!

3. Arranging pillows behind or under your tummy to relieve breathlessness can be very helpful.

Leg Cramps

Useful Asanas:

1. Salute to the Child #4, #8, and #10 (pp. 100–101, 104–106, 107)

2. All squatting postures

3. Foot Circles (p. 147)

4. Foot Rolls (p. 147)

Dietary Changes:

1. Increase calcium and potassium intake by including a banana, half a grapefruit, or an orange as a snack. Sesame seeds are high in calcium; sprinkle them on your salad.

2. Increase your calcium intake by including some of the following foods in your diet: cottage cheese, ice cream, yogurt, salmon, sardines, soybeans, almonds, sesame seeds. (See Chapter 3 for exact equivalents.)

Breathing and Relaxation Exercises:

While leg is cramped, inhale through the nose and exhale through a wide open mouth.

Cautions:

1. Do not stand in one place too long. Shift weight from one leg to the other.

2. Do not point your toes, point your heel instead.

Tips and Information:
1. Leg cramps are caused by the slowing of your blood circulation.
2. Walking one mile a day will help.
3. Elevate the legs higher than the heart to prevent cramps.
4. When you have a cramp, a hot water bottle or heating pad may help.
5. Putting pressure on the cramping area with your hands may bring relief.
6. Move your toes toward your knee and point your heel as you straighten your leg.

Nausea

Useful Asanas:
Chest Expansion (Standing) (pp. 94–96)

Dietary Changes:
1. Ten mg. per day of Vitamin B6 can help prevent nausea. Once nausea has started, use 25 mg. with each meal. Bananas are a good source of Vitamin B6.
2. Eat four to six small meals a day. Snack often.
3. Red Raspberry leaf, basil, ginger, or peppermint tea all help to eliminate nausea. Use one teaspoon of tea for one cup of hot water or use tea bags.
4. Keep some whole wheat crackers or dry whole wheat toast near your bed. Before getting up, eat the crackers and do a 15 minute Complete Relaxation. Then get up slowly.
5. Cold drinks such as ginger ale may help. Do not drink diet cola; it is high in caffein & salt.

Breathing and Relaxation Exercises:
Baby Breath (envision nausea moving down and out) (pp. 14–16)

Cautions:
1. Avoid coffee, and refined, greasy, or spicy foods.
2. Avoid highly acidic foods (such as orange juice) in the morning.
3. Do not go without eating or drinking because of nausea.
4. Do not drink diet cola soda because of its high caffeine and/or salt content.
5. If problem persists, speak to your doctor or midwife about it.

Tips and Information:
1. Nausea usually lasts the first trimester of pregnancy.
2. It is caused by a high estrogen level in your body and the rapid growth of your uterus.
3. Have faith that it will go away. Eventually it will.

Nasal congestion and nosebleeds

Useful Asanas and Cleansing Techniques:
1 Use a nasal wash with correct salt water solution to irrigate and clean nasal passages. Use as often as is needed. (p. 22)
2. Fish Position (pp. 117–119)

Dietary Changes:
1. Increase your intake of Vitamin C rich foods such as peppers, cabbage, oranges, lemons, grapefruits, strawberries, and broccoli.
2. Dairy products tend to be mucous producing. Supplement your diet with Dolomite, calcium and magnesium, or bone meal while decreasing dairy product consumption.

Breathing and Relaxation Exercises:
Alternate Nostril Breathing (at least five rounds very gently) (pp. 16–18)

Cautions:
Use nose drops or nasal sprays sparingly.

Tips and Information:
1. Increased blood volume often causes some capillaries to rupture and cause a nosebleed.
2. Lack of Vitamin C may be a contributing factor.
3. Vaseline in the tip of each nostril may help.
4. Stuffiness will disappear with the birth of the baby.
5. During pregnancy, inner nasal passages normally swell.

Stitch or soreness in rib area

Useful Asanas:
1. Chest Expansion (pp. 94–96)
2. Salute to the Child #2 and #11 (pp. 99, 108)

Breathing and Relaxation Exercises:
Mountain Breath (pp. 21–22)

Cautions:

Avoid Half Sit Up (in Basic Nine) and other postures which increase pressure on this area.

Tips and Information:

1. Often this disappears in the last six weeks of pregnancy once the baby drops into position to be born.
2. Change positions often.

Stretch Marks

Useful Asanas:

Salute to the Child (pp. 96–109) and the "Basic Nine" (pp. 79–96) help to keep skin in good tone.

Dietary Changes:

Keep your protein intake high and make sure you are eating foods from the four food groups daily.

Cautions:

Do not get depressed and think your tummy has turned into a road map!

Tips and Information:

1. Most pregnant women experience stretch marks. (You are in good company.)
2. Use naturally cold pressed vegetable oils such as sesame to keep your skin supple. Massage with oil your abdomen, hips, and any other area which seems to be stretching.
3. Light-haired people with very sensitive skin should oil and massage skin daily.
4. Red marks turn pale silver or white after the baby is born. They never completely disappear, but they become much less noticeable.

Swelling (Edema) (usually of hands and feet)

Useful Asanas:

1. Easy sitting posture (pp. 122–23)
2. Zen Sitting position (pp. 93)
3. Sitting on a Seiza bench (pp. 121–22)
4. Ankle Rotation, for swollen ankles (p. 147)
5. Leg Stretches Using a Wall (pp. 135–36)

Dietary Changes:
1. Do not eat highly salted foods such as potato chips, crackers, pretzels, salted peanuts, etc.
2. Do *not* eliminate salt from your diet. Keep salt consumption to a moderate level by preparing your own foods rather than using premixed, processed, or canned foods which are highly salted.
3. Eat a well-balanced diet, high in protein (See Chapter 3).

Breathing and Relaxation Exercises:
1. Deep Breathing with your legs on 45° angle against the wall for three to five minutes (pp. 134–35).
2. Mountain Breath (movement of hands may help eliminate some swelling) (pp. 21–22)

Cautions:
1. Tell your doctor about this condition as soon as you notice it. It can be the first stage of toxemia, which is a very serious disease of pregnancy.
2. Follow your doctor's or midwife's directions precisely.
3. Do not take diuretics (water pills) when you are pregnant.
4. Do not sit with a weight, such as another child, on your legs. This impedes your circulation.

Tips and Information:
1. A rise in estrogen in the body causes swelling in pregnancy. Some swelling is to be expected and is acceptable.
2. Hands, legs, and feet may get puffy and swollen. Remove your rings when you notice this condition. Do not wait, or the rings may have to be cut off!
3. Wear loose comfortable clothing.
4. Walking one mile a day helps to keep this condition under control.
5. Be sure to wear properly fitting shoes which may be larger than your normal size. Once the baby arrives, your feet will return to normal.

Varicose Veins

Useful Asanas:
1. Salute to the Child, #8 (pp. 104–6)
2. Basic Nine: Leg Lifts on the side (pp. 89–90)
3. Leg Cradles (pp. 83–84)
4. 45° Leg Rester (pp. 134–35)
5. Sitting on a Seiza Bench (pp. 121–22)

Breathing and Relaxation Exercises:

Complete Relaxation with legs elevated on two pillows, or on the seat part of a chair, or on a 45° angle against the wall. (pp. 152–55)

Cautions:

1. Do not wear restrictive socks (knee socks), garters, or belts.
2. Do not wear high-heeled shoes.
3. Do not stand for long periods of time.
4. Do not sit in cross-legged positions.

Tips and Information:

1. Varicose veins are enlarged veins close to the surface of the skin. They will usually disappear after the birth of the baby.
2. Walking one mile a day is very helpful.
3. Wear support hose if your doctor or midwife recommends them. Keep them near your bed and put them on before you get out of bed in the morning.
4. As often as you can, sit with your feet up higher than your heart.
5. Change positions frequently.

Five
The Many Moods
of Pregnancy

"I just don't feel like myself . . . I'm so moody. One moment I am crying and the next I may be laughing. Then there are days when I am even and calm. These moods swings are so unpredictable, I feel like I'm on an emotional roller coaster. Little things will bother me that I wouldn't have even thought about when I wasn't pregnant. However, I must say that I can empathize with people and events much more than I used to. The depths of my feelings is a new experience for me."

This description of the mood swings of pregnancy may or may not seem apt to you, for the emotional reactions that women experience during the waiting months are as varied as the women themselves. Many of my students have reported no noticeable change in their emotional state, while some have lived through new depths and intensities of emotion. Many women report a strong "nesting instinct" which imparts a feeling of calm. Although there is no definite pattern, it is important to know and accept the possibility of heightened emotions during your pregnancy. If you think about the physical and hormonal changes that naturally occur within your body as the baby develops, it is easily apparent that these changes will have some effect on your mental attitudes and emotions. Many times students have been awed by the sheer power of their emotions. Often, the kind of emotional control you had prior to your pregnancy is gone.

From a yogic point of view, all things within this universe contain life force or energy. When the female body is in the process of nurturing a new human being, the life force or vitality increases. The life force has a variety of names with which you may be familiar. Some of the most common are bioenergy, kundalini energy, vital life force, and inner energy. It is not important what you call this energy, only that you accept the fact that with the increase in the level of inner energy, there is often an increase in emotional reactions. This inner energy is the aspect of you which will exist forever, according to the yogic writings. When you are pregnant, you are really in a state of heightened vitality and life. You may be more sensitive to people, react more strongly to events, taste food with more clarity, or sense things before they happen. You are more alive!

You may be thinking at this moment, "If I am so much more alive, how come I am so tired and sleep so much?" That is a very valid question. There is a very definite difference between inner life force and the energy which we use for physical activities. Within the ancient yogic writings there is a description of a subtle body within our gross or physical body. There is no counterpart to this idea in modern western medicine. The subtle body contains the channels through which life force or bioenergy flows. From the bottom of your spine to the top of your head, there are seven energy centers or "chakras," each of which has a special relationship with a special inner realm and psychological function. (Fig. 5.1) The chakras can be thought of as the connectors between our inner nature and our physical body. With an increased output of inner energy, you may become more aware of the manifestations of the different chakras while you are pregnant.

The first chakra, located in the perineum, is called the root chakra and is concerned with the survival of the human body. The second chakra, located in the spine in the small of the back near the sexual area, is usually associated with sexual function. The third chakra, located in the spine just above the navel, is associated with the human drives of achieving power, fame, glory, and prestige. The fourth chakra, located in the spine behind the heart, is associated with love or compassion toward our fellow human beings. The fifth chakra, located in the spine at the base of the neck, is associated with communication, either speaking or writing. The sixth chakra, located between the eyebrows, is associated with seeing people as they really are, rather than how they pretend to be. The seventh chakra, located at the top of the head, is the connector point between energy within the body and energy outside of the body.

When inner energy flows through your inner channels, called "nadis," your perceptions and experiences in life change. This is extremely evident during pregnancy. For example, many women report feeling "protected" by a higher power or force during pregnancy. This is a very definite manifestation of the seventh chakra which is associated with a sense of spiritual awakening or awareness. Other women have been frightened by a sense of pressure in the head. This is a manifestation of the sixth and seventh chakra and can be easily remedied by "Alternate Nostril Breath" (p. 16–18). A feeling of pressure in the chest, as well as an increase in feelings of compassion, is related to the fourth chakra. The gut feelings in your stomach can be related to the lower chakras. Sometimes you may experience such deep emotions you can almost taste them. This is associated with the fifth chakra. Some mothers have visions of what their baby will look like, or be like, which later turn out to be accurate. This is a manifestation of the sixth chakra.

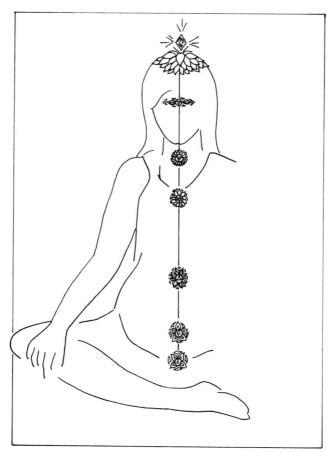

Figure 5.1 The seven *chakras* or energy centers of the body with their ancient symbols.

All of these characteristics of the chakras are simply indications of your higher potential and nature which becomes quite evident for some women during pregnancy. Often because the experiences are so vivid, you may begin to wonder about your sanity and, therefore, react in a negative way. Normally, you have two choices for dealing with heightened and turbulent emotions:

Retreat from the emotions, or *respond* to the emotions. However, during pregnancy the first choice is often eliminated, so you have to go with the second choice. Since most of your conditioning up to this point in your life has been along the lines of retreating from the emotion, you may have some difficulty at first adjusting to this new response. However, there are some helpful hints which can put all this theory to practical use. It is easy to say, "Oh, that's my fourth chakra getting energized," when you are crying bitterly over a TV episode. But when you are in a rage while your in-laws are visiting, it may be a much more difficult situation. The following plan of action for the many moods of pregnancy can be most useful to you:

1. Discuss your feelings openly with your mate. Talk about how the heightened emotions feel, how you feel helpless sometimes, how some emotional support would be most helpful, etc. Keep this dialogue going all through the pregnancy.

2. Keep a journal of your feelings. Use a small notebook to write out how you feel, why you think you feel that way, etc. Be honest about your feelings, writing down the negative ones as well. Try the "Turn the Leaf Over" (pp. 74–75) exercise in the journal as well as in your thinking processes.

3. Decide that you will go with your emotions. Suppressing your emotions will not be useful; often you may not be able to do it, then you feel guilty about not being able to do it, and a vicious cycle begins. Let the emotion ride over you and through you. Really *feel* love, hate, anger, fear, and depression. Imagine that you have a door at the top of your head and let the emotion ride all the way up your spine (that is the shortest route when you are in the later months) and out the door. Take two to three "Rock-the-Baby" breaths when the power of the emotion leaves.

4. Even if you feel lazy, practice your asanas as often as you can. The asanas within this book all stimulate and activate your inner energy to flow smoothly and freely along your inner passageways. That is why they are called asanas and not calisthenics. The asanas will help you to become calm and flexible while energizing you physically. One of my students remarked that she was very lazy and really did not want to practice, but she always felt better both mentally and physically after she did.

5. Practice calming breaths, such as Alternate Nostril Breath and Smooth Breath (pp. 16–18, 20–21). If you practice breathing for two to three minutes, it can change your whole perspective.

6. Practice Concentration or Meditation for 15–20 minutes twice a day on a regular basis. (See Chapter 9, for specific details.)

7. Share your emotions mentally with the baby. Since the baby is feeling the result of those emotions while living inside your agitated or depressed body, you may as well have a mental discussion about it. Be honest with the baby. Being angry is just as much a part of motherhood as being loving. Children seem to instinctively understand this. An incident comes to mind which will illustrate my point. For some reason which I cannot recall, I had yelled at my older son, Mathew, who was about five years old at the time. He already knew how to write, so he went to his room, made the following note, and gave it to me: "I still love you even when your (sic) mad." I still have that note, for the message was one we all need to remember from time to time.

8. Accept your heightened sensitivity as nature's way of preparing you for your forthcoming motherhood role. You will need heightened ESP to know how to communicate with a screaming baby who is not hungry or sleepy at 3:00 A.M. Accepting and going with the situation rather than fighting it can be a valuable part of training for motherhood.

9. During times of extremely heightened emotions, you may forget to eat, or may eat whatever is handy (cookies, soda, etc.). If you are feeling extremely depressed, you may indulge in a variety of junk foods which you think will help you feel better. Emotional states (very quickly) burn up the B vitamins which are in your body. Since the body cannot manufacture B vitamins and is, therefore, dependent on your diet for a good supply, you must be very aware of what you are eating. By getting into the habit of snacking on B vitamin rich foods such as sunflower, pumpkin, or sesame seeds, you should not experience depression due to a lack of these vitamins. Although B vitamins play a part in emotional stability, only a balanced diet chosen wisely from the four main food groups will ensure physical and mental well being. Remember to eat five or six small meals a day to minimize nausea as well as emotional upsets.

One very pleasant aspect of the old ideas about pregnancy still persists. You may find that people open doors for you, carry packages, or just treat you a bit special when you are pregnant. Enjoy this special treatment, for most of it will shift over to the baby, immediately after the birth. Blend this special treatment with a mental attitude of increased inner vitality, increased health, increased creativity, and new life. Allow yourself to be open to many new experiences which can be yours during the waiting months.

Six

Fear Is
a Four-Letter Word

Of all the topics discussed in my classes, none is more consistent than the fears associated with pregnancy, birth, and motherhood. Where do these fears come from?

Maybe your mother talked to you about her negative birth experience. Maybe it was your best friend questioning her ability to cope. In any event, it really does not matter where you first acquired these fears. It is, however, most important that you *now* become aware of your fears and do something to allay them.

"What are your biggest fears during pregnancy?" My students usually respond to this question with silence. Everyone looks around; no one wants to admit she is fearful. Then some brave soul quietly verbalizes her fear about not having a normal child. Quickly, the group becomes very vocal. One student usually says, "Oh, you have that fear too?" As soon as it becomes obvious that the primary fears during pregnancy are fairly universal, everyone sighs with relief. Then we can get to the real reasons for the discussion.

"What should you do with your fears?" is usually the next question raised. Throughout the ensuing discussion, it becomes apparent that sharing your fears with a group in the same situation helps make those fears diminish or in some cases disappear.

One conclusion which is often reached during these talks relates to facing your fears. We have found that *not* facing your fears headlong can produce pain and suffering, while doing the opposite—leveling with yourself and the group—helps eradicate the fear. The group is always happy to find out that 95% of all babies born in this country at the present time are perfectly normal. The odds are certainly in your favor!

This leads to a second, very important, point: most fear thrives in ignorance. Many fears are based on your imaginary understanding of a situation rather than a factual one. If, for example, a student is afraid of being in the hospital, I usually advise a tour of the local hospital to see all the areas which she may be using for labor, birth, and confinement. If the hospital is still not agreeable to her, then she and her husband might explore the idea of home birth. The options are there, but first you must know what you are fighting.

Another extremely important point that usually emerges from these group discussions is that help is available in most instances when you really need it. I continually emphasize in my classes that the pregnant woman will be helped. She may have to ask very loudly for what she wants at special times, but in most cases she and her baby will be helped. When my students accept the idea that they will be helped when they need it, many of their fears disappear.

Worrying, rather than dealing with fear, makes the emotion grow totally out of proportion. Many women spend their whole pregnancy worrying that this or that will go wrong. What a waste of energy! Use these nine months to develop physically, mentally, and emotionally for the child to come.

Yoga can help you learn to be totally aware of your feelings and experiences during the waiting time. Once your fears are recognized, you should talk about them. "Great," you may say, "but I don't happen to have a class or group to talk to." Remember that there are always people to talk to. Perhaps you can talk with your husband, doctor, midwife, or a friend.

The positive experience of sharing time and feelings with other pregnant women seems to help allay fears. One of the most beneficial parts of my class, "Yoga for the Mother-To-Be," is the socializing that goes on between women in the same situation. Find out if there is a group like this in your area. Perhaps you could start your own informal group.

Learning to recognize, admit, and face your feelings will make your pregnancy a more positive experience. There is a very simple mental exercise which is a form of yoga concentration that is most beneficial for dealing with your fears once you have pinpointed them. This mental exercise is called "Turn Over the Leaf."

Imagine: Each one of your fears is a leaf with two very different sides:

Side 1: FEAR		Side 2: FAITH
On this leaf you find: "I will never be able to make it through labor and delivery."	TURN IT OVER	On the other side you will find: "I will have the inner strength and help I need to have a good birth experience."

Or: "I will not be able to take care of the baby once it arrives."	TURN IT OVER	"I am going to educate myself by reading books and talking to other new mothers. I may not have all the answers, but I will do the best I can."
Or: "I will not be able to cope with all the new responsibilities."	TURN IT OVER	"I have faith in myself and I know I can do a good job. I will get help when I need it."

Every time you notice your head filled with fears about the baby or your new motherhood role, you have to remember to turn over the leaf. With some practice, you can learn not to be drawn into the power of negative thoughts, but to turn them over to see their positive aspects. The most rewarding benefit of this mental exercise is a better understanding of the workings of your brain.

Your mental attitude helps to create the inner environment for your child. The baby shares your body, and experiences many of your feelings. This exercise, in addition to the Pregnancy Concentrations in Chapter 10, will help you to stay in a positive frame of mind during your pregnancy. A positive attitude will contribute to your enjoyment, as well as your mate's and your baby's enjoyment, of this new adventure in your lives.

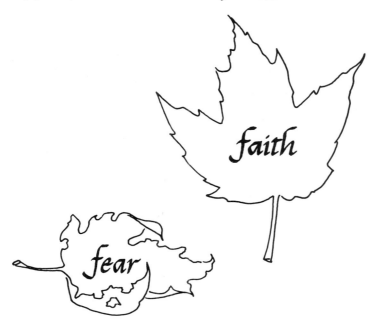

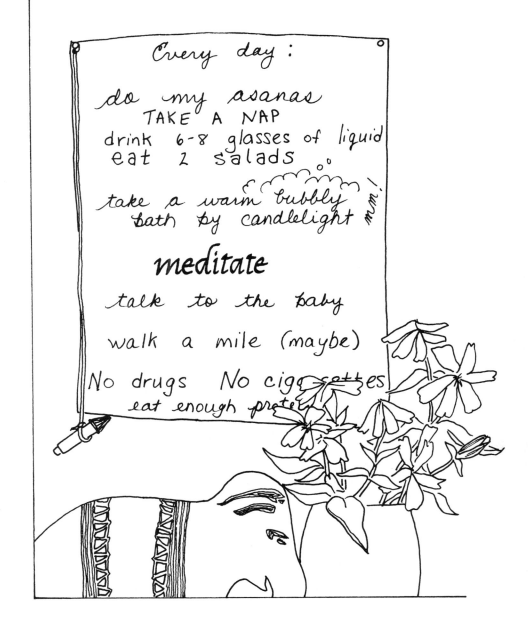

Every day :

do my asanas
TAKE A NAP
drink 6-8 glasses of liquid
eat 2 salads

take a warm bubbly
bath by candlelight mm!

meditate

talk to the baby

walk a mile (maybe)

No drugs   No cigarettes
eat enough protein

Seven

Asanas for All the Pregnant Months

A: PRACTICE GUIDELINES

During pregnancy your body is constantly changing and growing on the inside. Therefore, the exercises you do on the outside have to change and adapt to your growing shape and weight. Many of the exercises you may have done before the advent of the baby can be continued all during the pregnant months, with the agreement of your doctor or midwife. When and if these forms of exercise become uncomfortable or straining to you, they should be minimized or eliminated completely. A brisk daily one-mile walk can be easily substituted for the more strenuous exercises.

The idea that doing nothing physically for nine months because you are in a "delicate condition" is no longer fashionable or acceptable. In fact, it is becoming more evident that a total exercise and relaxation program throughout the full nine months of pregnancy often facilitates a more positive, easier, and often shorter birth experience. You will find that you will feel better after you have begun to practice some yoga asanas.

For your convenience, a set of "Basic Nine" exercises has been developed; these postures should be the backbone of your exercise program. All nine postures can and should be used throughout the pregnancy. Also included here is a creative series of 12 interwoven positions called "Salute to the Child," which is safe during *all* the pregnant months. It is advisable to use the Rock-the-Baby Breath (pp. 13–14) or Baby Breath (pp. 14–16) during your practice sessions. What follows are some basic instructions for doing all the exercises.

1. Take one or two "Rock-the-Baby" or "Baby Breaths."
2. Slowly assume chosen position. Relax any muscles you are not directly stretching.
3. Hold and stretch, trying to be still for as long as is comfortable.
4. Slowly return to starting position.
5. Take one or two "Rock-the-Baby" or "Baby Breaths."
6. Follow with another asana or a Relaxation position and more breathing.
7. *Keep your mental awareness at all times on the physical feelings of all your movements, on your breathing, or on your baby.*

If you disregard these directions and race through the asanas, thinking about what you will make for dinner or what you are going to do next week, all of your efforts will be for very little benefit and may, in fact, do you some harm. To make these postures work for you, they must be done *slowly* with total concentration. The unifying of your mind, body, and breath will ensure success with the program and a more positive, rewarding pregnancy.

GUIDELINES FOR PRACTICING PRENATAL YOGA

1. *Always* check with your doctor or midwife before beginning any exercise program.
2. *Always* try to be consistent with your practice times (20–30 minutes per day is fine).
3. *Always* wear loose comfortable clothing (leotards are not necessary.)
4. *Always* practice on a comfortable mat, such as a piece of indoor/outdoor carpeting.
5. *Always* practice sitting cross-legged and squatting daily.
6. *Always* move slowly from one position to another.
7. *Always* take two to three "Rock-the-Baby" or "Baby Breaths" between every position.

1. *Never* get into pain while practicing.
2. *Never* rush through a practice session.
3. *Never* exercise in a poorly ventilated room.
4. *Never* practice right after eating. Wait at least one to two hrs.
5. *Never* practice inverted postures (Shoulderstand, Plough, Headstand) unless you are an experienced practitioner.
6. *Never* do regular sit-ups.
7. *Never* do strenuous upward stretching or forward bending postures.
8. *Never* wear shoes while practicing.

8. *Always* keep your mind on what you are feeling as you stretch and relax.

9. *Always* stretch as far as you can comfortably and then relax into the stretch.

10. *Always* end your practice session with several abdominal breaths and a Complete Relaxation.

9. *Never* do postures which involve violent stomach contractions.

10. *Never* do postures lying flat on your stomach (Cobra, Bow, and Locust).

If you follow these simple rules, you will find that you will begin to look forward to your practice time. The practice cassette tapes which are listed in the appendix may be helpful to induce you to practice. If you use the same practice mat each day, seeing it will remind you to do your yoga. Declare 20 or 30 minutes each day your private time. Take the phone off the hook; tune out the world for a short time. You'll find that you emerge from this time feeling refreshed and renewed.

B: "THE BASIC NINE"

The core of your prenatal exercise routine should be the "Basic Nine." Each exercise will benefit your body in a special way, but all the exercises will release tension and tiredness from your body and your mind. Spend some time early in your pregnancy learning these simple and enjoyable exercises and you will be rewarded with a more trouble-free pregnancy. Remember that as your body grows larger, you will have to make certain changes and allowances while practicing. Do not become discouraged when an exercise which seemed relatively easy in the fifth month becomes more difficult in the eighth or ninth month.

1A: Neck Rolls

This should be practiced in any comfortable sitting position.

Benefits:
· Relieves pain and tension in the neck
· Keeps your neck and shoulders loose and limber
· Helps to relax the entire body, eliminate insomnia, and prevent headaches

Directions:

1. In any comfortable sitting position, let your head fall loosely forward with your chin near your chest, while you close your eyes. Relax your facial muscles as completely as possible. (Figure 7B.1)

2. Keeping your shoulders still, very slowly roll your head around to your right side (right ear near right shoulder). Let the weight of your head pull your neck muscles. (Figure 7B.2)

3. Continue to move your head very slowly around until it hangs back. (Figure 7B.3) Keep your mouth loose and open as if you were a bit tipsy.

4. Continue around toward your left side and finally back to your forward position. (Figure 7B.4)

5. Now reverse directions and rotate your head to the left.

6. Repeat two to three times in each direction taking at least 20 seconds for one rotation. Make your circles even and smooth.

7. When you have finished, slowly shift your head up straight and take two to three deep breaths.

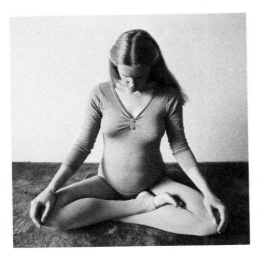

Figure 7B.1   Neck Roll with head forward.

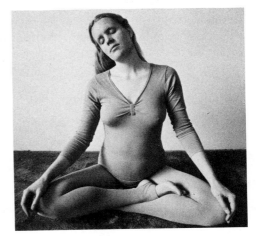

Figure 7B.2   Neck Roll with head to the right.

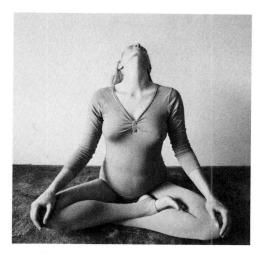

Figure 7B.3 Neck Roll with head hanging back.

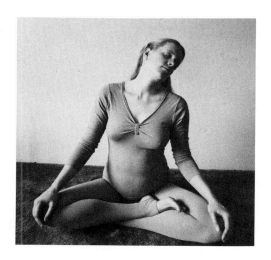

Figure 7B.4 Neck Roll with head to the left.

Cautions and Comments:

- Your neck may crack and creak. You are not falling apart! This is perfectly normal and helpful for keeping the neck area—a very popular tension spot—loose and limber.

- Practice this exercise during TV commercials or during other spare moments in the day.

- You can inhale as you move your head half way around and exhale the other half of the neck roll.

- This exercise is especially helpful for women who work in offices and are bending forward all day.

- Neck rolls are excellent as a quick energizer.

1B.   Neck Twists

These can be practiced either sitting or standing.

Benefits:
- Releases tension in the shoulders and the neck
- Helps to prevent or eliminate double chin
- Increases body flexibility

Directions:
1. Shift your head to the center and up straight.
2. Move your head as far around to the right side as you can comfortably. Look over your right shoulder and in back of you. Imagine that your favorite movie star is in back of you and you are stretching to see him. (Figure 7B.5)
3. When you have twisted your head around as far as you can, relax your shoulders and the muscles in your neck and face. Then twist a bit farther. Hold for 15–20 seconds or as long as is comfortable.
4. Return to the center and repeat the same movements on the other side.
5. Return your head to the center and take two to three "Rock-the-Baby" or "Baby Breaths." Repeat three more times.

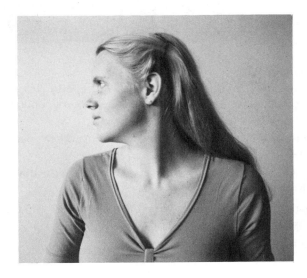

Figure 7B.5
Neck Twist.

Cautions and Comments:
- This exercise is very easy to practice in the supermarket.
- If you are working in an office, practice this movement three to four times a day.
- Do not twist so far that you get into pain.
- Remember to keep your shoulders relaxed throughout this exercise.

2. Leg Cradles

Benefits:
- Limbers the legs, hips, and pelvic area so that you can more comfortably sit in a cross-legged position
- Loosens tight muscle sets in your thighs and calves
- Prepares the legs for the pushing stage of labor
- Strengthens your arms and shoulders while releasing tension

Directions:
1. Sit in a comfortable cross-legged position with your back unsupported, and your head and shoulders up straight.
2. Place your right foot in the crook of your left elbow while you wrap your right arm around the outside of the right leg. Clasp your hands in front of your leg if you can. (Figure 7B.6) If that is impossible, simply hold your right foot with the left hand and right knee with the right hand.

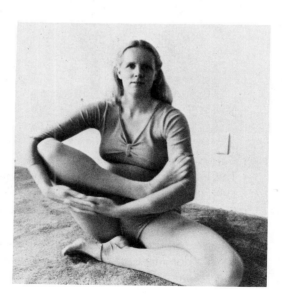

Figure 7B.6
Leg Cradles.

3. Move the cradled leg from side to side four to five times.

4. Stretch the right foot forward and make a slow circular motion with it to stretch your shoulders as well as your right leg. Repeat four to five times.

5. Place your left hand on the floor behind you with your fingers facing away from your body.

6. Place your *right* hand either on the inside bottom arch of the *right* foot or on the ankle or calf area of the right leg while you straighten out your leg. (Figure 7B.7)

7. Move the leg from side to side as far as is comfortable for you. Repeat four to five times.

8. When you become fatigued, bring the leg down and back into a cross-legged position.

9. Take two to three "Rock-the-Baby" breaths and repeat on other side.

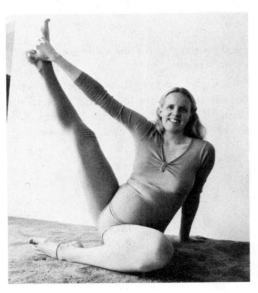

Figure 7B.7 Outstretched Leg Movement.

Cautions and Comments:

- This exercise may seem difficult when you first practice it, but in time, you will notice your legs getting more limber and loose.

- Keep your knee bent a bit during section #6 of this exercise if it is painful to straighten out your leg.

- One leg may be much easier to exercise than the other. We tend to have a dominant leg as well as a dominant arm.

- This exercise can be easily practiced during TV commercials.

3. Pregnancy Spinal Twist

This can be practiced sitting cross-legged or sitting in a chair.

Benefits:

- Keeps the sides of your growing waistline intact
- Keeps your spine limber and, thereby, has a therapeutic effect on your nervous system
- Relieves tension and realigns your vertebrae
- Is an energizing posture for a quick pick-up

Directions:

1. Sitting up straight in a cross-legged position, place your left hand on your right knee.
2. Stretch your right arm directly to the right side and then bring as far behind you as possible.
3. Place the right hand down on the mat behind you with your fingers pointing away from your body. Be sure your hand is as close to your body as is possible.
4. Turn your head and look over your right shoulder.
5. Relax the shoulders, facial muscles, and the extended arm and twist a bit further. (Figure 7B.8)

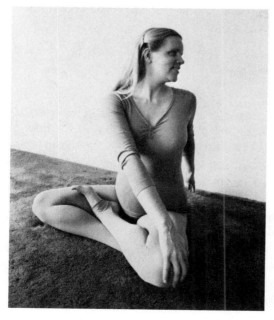

Figure 7B.8 Pregnancy Spinal Twist.

6. Hold for 10–20 seconds or until you are fatigued and then return to starting position.

7. Take two to three "Rock-the-Baby" breaths and repeat the same movements on the left side. Repeat movements twice more.

Cautions and Comments:
- Once you have placed your hand on the floor in back of you, do not tip backwards. Move your hand closer to you for better balance.
- To increase the twist, you can bend your front arm and pull your front shoulder closer to the front opposite knee.
- It takes time to learn to relax into this posture, but its benefits will be increased if you take the time.
- Always remember to twist in both directions for an even stretch.

4. The Bridge with Preparatory Pelvic Rocking

This should be practiced on your back with your knees bent and your feet flat on your mat.

Benefits:
- Limbers the spine and makes it flexible
- It is very helpful for eliminating or minimizing pregnancy backache
- Tones the central nervous system
- Relieves neck strain
- Tones and tightens the thighs

Directions:
1. Lying flat on your back, separate both legs a comfortable distance apart. Bend both your knees and place both feet flat on the floor as close to your body as you can. Keep your hands at your sides.
2. *Exhale* and flatten your lower back down to the mat. *Inhale* and raise *just* the lower back up off the mat. Keep your buttocks on the mat. (Figures 7B.9 and 7B.10)
3. Repeat this Pelvic Rocking five to ten times coordinating your breathing with your pelvic movements.
4. Once your lower back begins to feel warm, then begin to raise your torso into the air. (Figure 7B.11)

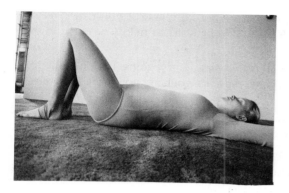

Figure 7B.9 Pelvic Rock with spine lowered.

Figure 7B.10 Pelvic Rock with spine raised.

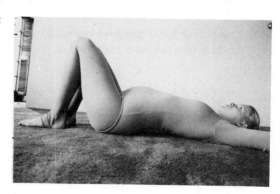

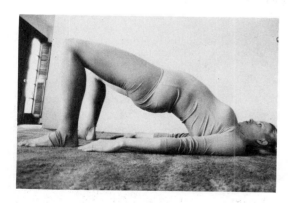

Figure 7B.11
The Completed Bridge.

5. Push your torso and your baby up a bit higher if you can. You may want to put your hands around your waist to help you push up even higher.

6. For an extra stretch you may want to try going up on your toes. (Figure 7B.12) Relax all the muscles you are not using and stretch into the asana.

7. Hold for 15–30 seconds while breathing normally. Keep your mental concentration on your breathing, bodily feelings, or your baby.

8. Control your descent by coming down one vertebra at a time.

9. You may want to follow the Bridge with the Lower Back Rocker if you feel any strain in the lower back.

10. To do the Lower Back Rocker, bring both knees on either side of the baby and wrap your hands around your knees and rock side to side for a while. (Figure 7B.13)

11. Once you have finished rocking, place your hands and feet in the starting position and take two to three ''Rock-the-Baby'' breaths.

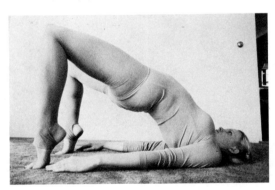

Figure 7B.12 The Bridge on the toes.

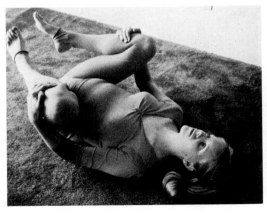

Figure 7B.13 The Lower Back Rocker.

Cautions and Comments:
- Many pregnant women love this exercise because it releases lower back tension and eliminates pain in that area.
- At the very first sign of a backache, this is the posture to practice. Do it several times.
- As your back strengthens, you may find you do not need to use your hands to push up higher.
- Placing your hands on your ankles before going up will give you a stronger stretch. This hand position becomes difficult in the later months.
- If you have been experiencing leg cramps, be careful with the Bridge variation on your toes for you may develop more cramps.

5. Side Leg Circles with a Half Bow

This should be practiced lying comfortably on your side.

Benefits:
- Loosens the entire pelvic area
- Helps to drain excess blood out of the legs
- Helps to relieve lower backache
- Tones and keeps the legs shapely
- Firms the arms and strengthens the shoulders
- Often the Half Bow will help to relieve round ligament (lower groin) cramps

Directions:
1. Lie on your left side, legs together, your left arm outstretched with your head leaning on it. (You can also raise your head and support it with your left palm covering your ear.)
2. Put your right hand on the floor near your chest for support. Bend your left leg for better balance.
3. Raise the top leg up into the air as high as you can. You may want to support the right thigh with your right hand.
4. Make 10 rotations with your right foot only, five in each direction.
5. Once the ankle feels loose and warm, start to make circles with the entire leg. Make small circles which keep increasing in size as you rotate your leg. (Figure 7B.14)
6. When your leg feels fatigued, lower it and take two to three "Rock-the-Baby" breaths.

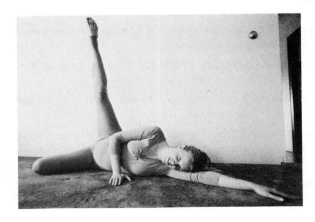

Figure 7B.14 Leg Circles on the side.

7. Now bend the top right leg, reach back, and grab onto your right ankle with your right hand.

8. Keeping your right arm straight, pull the right foot far behind you as you open up the right leg. (Figure 7B.15)

9. Hold this stretch for 15–30 seconds or as long as comfortable and then lower and relax by taking two to three "Rock-the-Baby" or "Baby Breaths."

10. Roll over and repeat both sets of movements on the other side.

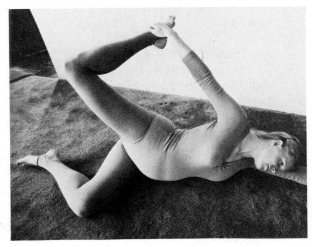

Figure 7B.15 The Side Bow.

Cautions and Comments:

• When making leg circles, start with small ones but end with the largest circles you can make. This is very important for keeping the pelvic area loose and moveable for the birthing process.

• When practicing the Half Bow, be sure to keep your top arm straight for a maximum stretch. If you feel a tight pull across your abdomen, lower the bent leg a bit to minimize the pull.

• Resting your head on your hand during the Half Bow may be more comfortable for you.

• During the later months, you may have to do fewer leg circles. Often the hip joints become more sensitive as the pregnancy progresses.

6.   Pregnancy Sit-Up

This should be practiced on your back with your knees bent and your feet flat on the floor.

Benefits:

• Prepares the abdominal oblique muscles for the pushing stage of labor

• Gently strengthens your lower back, arms and shoulders

• Keeps your buttocks tight and firm

Directions:

1. Lie on your back with your knees bent and your feet on the floor about eight to ten inches apart.

2. Raise both arms, palms together or hands clasped, above your chest. (Figure 7B.16)

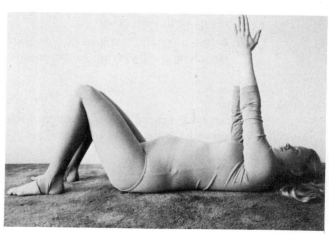

Figure 7B.16 Preparation for the Pregnancy Sit-Up.

3. Roll towards the right, raising your head and shoulders and stretch both hands on the outside of your right knee. (Figure 7B.17)

4. Hold, breathing normally, 15–30 seconds or for as long as comfortable.

5. Come back to a starting position. Take a breath.

6. Repeat on the other side. Repeat each side two to five times taking two to three "Rock-the-Baby" breaths between each Pregnancy Sit-Up.

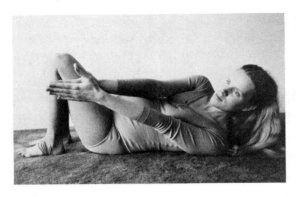

Figure 7B.17 The Pregnancy Sit-Up.

Cautions and Comments:
- Keep breathing while you are holding the Sit-Up. *Do not hold your breath.*
- This exercise may grow progressively more difficult as the end of the pregnancy nears. You should cut down the number of repetitions you do, but do not stop practicing it.
- When you are pushing your baby into this level of awareness and your body works perfectly, you will personally experience the dividends of this exercise.
- As the pregnancy progresses, you should rock more to the side before stretching the hands up to the outside of your knees.

7. Anal Lock

This can be practiced in any position. Preferable positions are Zen Sitting Position or lying flat on your back.

Benefits:
- Massages and tones the female sex organs
- Highly beneficial for the nerves and organs of the reproductive system
- Helps to prevent constipation and hemorrhoids
- Keeps the sexual area responsive while preparing the birth canal area for your baby's birth

Directions:

1. Sit in the Zen Sitting Position with your buttocks on your heels (Figure 7B.18). If this is not comfortable for your ankles, shift both feet over to your right side next to your right hip.

2. Inhale smoothly and slowly.

3. As you exhale, contract the buttocks, thereby contracting the anal, vaginal, and urethral muscles. Hold this contraction during your exhalation, but do not hold your breath.

4. Inhale and relax the pelvic floor muscles.

5. Repeat five to ten times.

6. Relax and take two to three "Rock-the-Baby" breaths.

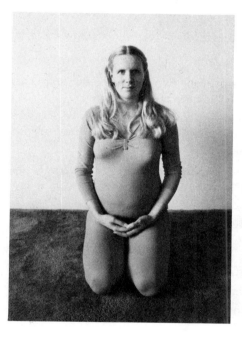

Figure 7B.18 Zen Sitting Position for the Anal Lock.

Cautions and Comments:

• With some practice you can learn to contract and release only the anal muscles, only the vaginal muscles, or only the bladder muscles. This takes time and effort.

• Do this exercise while you are at work, two to three times during the day.

• This posture can also be practiced in a flat back lying position, with your ankles crossed. You may choose to practice the Anal Lock in a back lying position until the later months of pregnancy when this position often becomes uncomfortable and unsafe.

- This posture or the Pelvic Floor Exercises (Sexercises) should be practiced right after the birth of the baby to help promote quick healing of the birth canal.

8. Chest Expansion or Support for the "Milk Factory"

This should be practiced while standing but can be practiced in a chair.

Benefits:
- Relieves tension in the neck, shoulders, and upper back while strengthening these areas
- Develops and strengthens the muscle groups which support the breasts
- Is a quick energizer
- Expands your lungs and chest area for increased breathing capacity

Directions:
1. Standing straight with your feet even, two to three feet apart, get your weight evenly distributed. Tuck the buttocks under.
2. With your arms hanging loosely at your sides, push your shoulder blades together. Breathe normally; hold for a count of five; release.
3. Take one "Rock-the-Baby" breath.
4. Bring your hands behind you and clasp them together, (palms facing inward) keeping your arms as straight as you can.
5. Pushing your shoulder blades together, lift your arms up as close to your head as possible. Breathe normally as you hold for five to 30 seconds. (Figure 7B.19)
6. Bend from the waist, keeping your head up while you keep your arms in the same position. Hold for five to thirty seconds. (Figure 7B.20)
7. Straighten up, keeping your hands clasped.
8. Relax your shoulders and arms as you take two to three "Rock-the-Baby" breaths.
9. Turn your right foot at a 90° angle and bend it at the knee.
10. Bend and stretch over the bent knee keeping your chin up while your arms are being stretched up toward your head. Hold for five to 30 seconds. (Figure 7B.21)
11. Straighten up and return to the center. Take two to three "Rock-the-Baby" breaths.
12. Repeat the same movement on the other side.
13. When you have finished, take two to three "Rock-the-Baby" breaths.

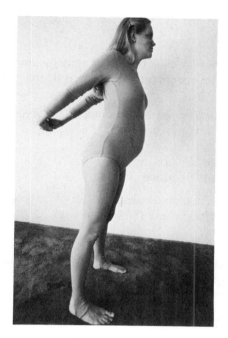

Figure 7B.19 Chest Expansion standing straight.

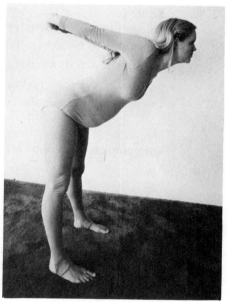

Figure 7B.20 Chest Expansion with forward bend.

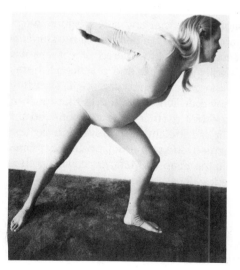

Figure 7B.21 Chest Expansion to the side.

Cautions and Comments:
- It may be advisable to do this exercise next to a chair at the beginning, for you have to develop your concentration to balance in the third movement to the side.
- To increase the stretch across your chest and shoulders, try Steps 4–7 with your palms touching and thumbs together.

9.   Complete Relaxation:
the most Important Exercise of All!

This can be practiced flat on your back until the seventh month of pregnancy, then lying on your left or right side in any comfortable position.

Benefits:
- Releases tension by deeply relaxing the muscles and the nervous system
- Trains you to be able to completely relax at will
- Restores peace of mind
- Mastery of this exercise can shorten your laboring time by up to 45%
- Deepens your conscious connection with your future baby

Directions:
See complete directions on pp. 155–57.

C: SALUTE TO THE CHILD

The "Salute to the Child" is an innovative concept in prenatal yoga. It evolved, quite naturally, from a number of highly beneficial and safe postures which can be practiced all during the pregnant months. One day one of my students, who had been studying yoga for several years, wondered why there was not a set of asanas which she could easily remember and practice each day. She had been practicing "Salute to the Sun" (a popular yogic stretching series) daily prior to her pregnancy; however, when she found that much of the Sun Salutation was unsafe for expectant mothers, she discontinued this routine. I found the idea of a series of linked stretches very novel and exciting. My mother-to-be classes and I experimented with numerous posture combinations, finally developing the series within this chapter. Many expectant mothers have worked with and enjoyed this series since its inception.

By incorporating this series of interwoven postures into your daily practice routine, you should continue to feel limber and energetic throughout your pregnancy. This series will prepare your body both physically and mentally for the birth experience. Study the /hotos, line drawings, and instructions until you feel familiar with the movements. During each position, first feel the particular stretches; second, focus in on your future child for a few seconds and then go on to the next position. Some positions require more deep breathing between them than others. Try out Salute to the Child and see how much better you feel once you have completed the series!

1. Standing Prayer Pose
2. Shoulder Blade Stretch: Front to Back
3. The Cradle Stretch
4. Squat with Baby Breath
5. Butterfly with Breath Coordination
6. Spinal Twist in "Z" Sitting Position
7. Cat Position
8. Leg Stretches in Cat Position
9. Arm Stretches in Zen Sitting Position
10. Stretching Out of a Squat
11. Modified Backward Bend
12. Standing Prayer Pose

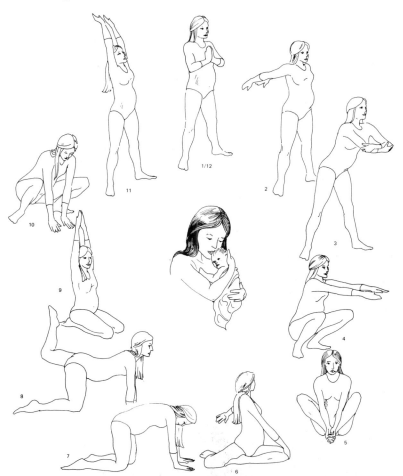

Figure 7C.1 The twelve poses of Salute to the Child.

Salute to the Child

This should be practiced one to three times daily.

Benefits:
- Prepares the correct muscle sets throughout your body for the rigors of birth
- Keeps your spine and body flexible and supple, which benefits your nervous system
- Develops your concentration skills
- Preserves and tones those parts of your body which are not directly affected by the pregnancy
- Keeps the pregnant body supple and relaxed
- Helps to foster a more direct connection between you and your baby
- Releases tensions for a heightened feeling of peace and relaxation

Directions:
Position 1: Standing Prayer Pose
1. Stand up straight with your feet at a 45° angle outward and 12–16 inches apart.
2. Place your hands, palms together, next to your breast bone. Take one to two "Rock-the-Baby" breaths as you become centered. Let tranquility and stillness fill you as you inhale, and nervousness and tiredness leave you as you exhale. (Figure 7C.2)

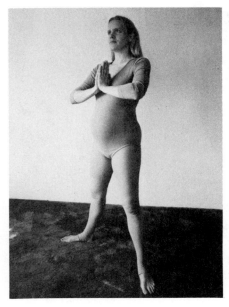

Figure 7C.2 Standing Prayer Pose.

Position 2: Shoulder Blade Stretch—Front to Back

1. Stretch your arms directly out in front of you, palms together, while you focus on the stretching feeling across your shoulders. (Figure 7C.3)

2. Twist the arms so that your palms face upward. Hold five seconds, then bring your arms behind you shoulder distance apart. (Figure 7C.4)

3. Arch your chest and baby area forward as you gently push your shoulder blades together. Hold this position five to ten seconds, breathing normally.

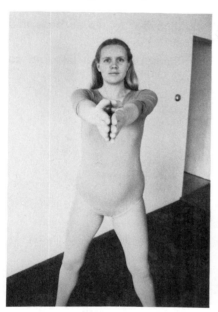

Figure 7C.3   Shoulder Blade Stretch in front.

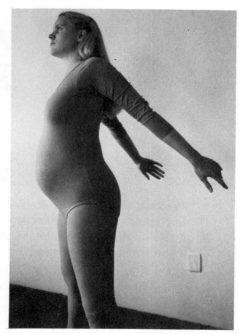

Figure 7C.4   Shoulder Blade Stretch in back.

Position 3: The Cradle Stretch

1. Release the arms and bring them directly in front of your chest. Place the right hand on the left elbow and the left hand on the right elbow.

2. Bend slightly forward and feel as if your arms and upper back are being stretched. Hold this position for five to ten seconds, breathing normally.

3. Holding your arms in this same position, turn as far to the right as you can. Hold, breathing normally for five to ten seconds. (Figure 7C.5)

4. Repeat movement to the left side holding five to ten seconds and breathing normally.

5. Return to the center, letting the arms hang down and take one to two "Rock-the-Baby" breaths.

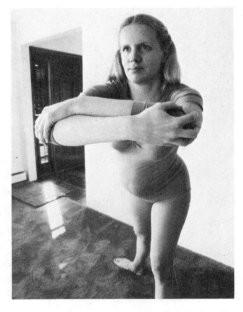

Figure 7C.5 The Cradle Stretch.

Position 4: Squat with Baby Breath

1. Stretching your arms directly in front of you palms down, begin to go into a squatting position. Bend your knees over your feet and assume a squat, either on your toes or on flat feet. (Figure 7C.6)

2. Place your hands on the mat between your feet to get your balance. Once balanced, put your elbows on your knees and your palms together.

3. Keeping your head up, take a "Baby Breath" in this position imagining that the air is coming into your navel directly to your baby and is being exhaled out of your wide open birth canal. Push down and slightly forward with the vaginal muscles as you exhale. Keep your awareness on the area through which your baby will have to pass in order to be born. (Figure 7C.7)

4. If comfort permits (and after some practice, it will . . .), do a second "Baby Breath." *Note:* If you have varicose veins, do not do the Baby Breaths in this position. Immediately proceed to 5.

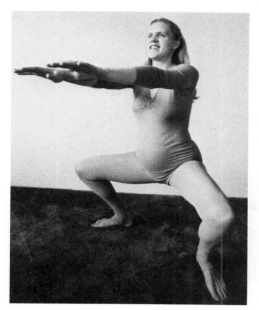

Figure 7C.6   Going into a Squat.

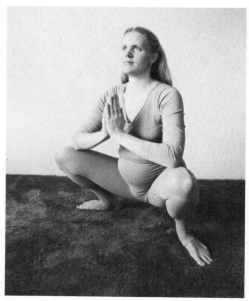

Figure 7C.7   A Squat with Baby Breath.

Position 5: The Butterfly with Breath Coordination

1. Place your hands on the mat in back of you for support as you bring your buttocks down to the mat.

2. Shift your legs so that your knees are out to the sides and the soles of your feet are touching. Clasp your hands and place them on your toes.

3. Inhale as you bring your knees up as close to your arms as you can. Exhale as you lower your knees as close to the mat as you can. (Figure 7C.8)

4. Repeat four to five times trying to get your knees even closer to the mat each time. Feel the stretch in the inner thigh and knee areas.

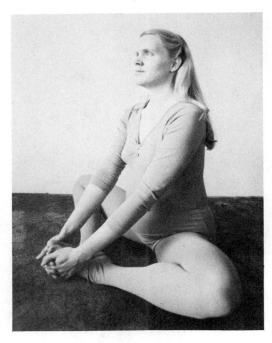

Figure 7C.8 Butterfly with breath coordination.

Position 6: Spinal Twist in a "Z" Sitting Position

1. Keeping your left knee in the same outward position, move your right knee next to your left heel. This is the "Z" sitting position.

2. Place your right hand on your left knee while you extend your left hand out straight on the left side.

3. Move your extended left arm as far behind you as you can comfortably and look over your left shoulder toward the outstretched arm. (Figure 7C.9)

Figure 7C.9 Spinal Twist in "Z" sitting position.

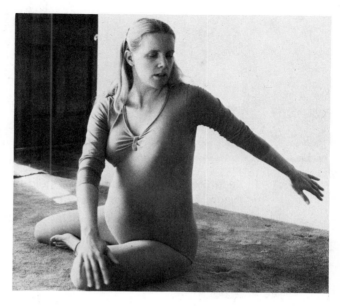

4. Hold five to 30 seconds, breathing normally as you begin to relax into this twisting posture. Relax your shoulders, your facial muscles, and your neck; twist around a bit more. (For increased stretch, imagine your favorite movie star is standing right behind you and you have to twist around to see him. Keep twisting and relaxing to see him better!)

5. Move back to your starting position in the center, placing your hands in your lap as you take two "Rock-the-Baby" breaths.

6. Next, place your left hand on your right knee and repeat the same movements on the right side. Hold the twist on the right five to 30 seconds breathing normally and then return to center.

7. Optional Twist: Reverse your leg positions and twist once in each direction holding and relaxing into each position five to ten seconds and breathing normally. Remember to relax into each twist for maximum tension-releasing benefits.

Position 7: Cat Position

1. Slide your hands along your thighs and then on to the mat while raising your buttocks into the air and assuming a cat position. (Figure 7C.10)

2. Place your hands and feet the same distance apart; stretch your back up as high as you can, feeling a stretch to your spine, arms, and hands. Your chin will naturally move closer to your chest.

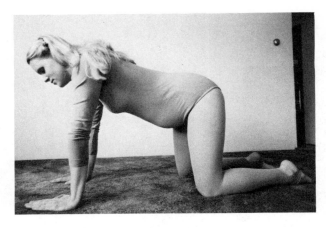

Figure 7C.10 The Cat with a flat back.

3. Keep breathing normally as you hold this stretch five to ten seconds (Figure 7C.11) and then return to a flat back position.
4. Take one to two "Rock-the-Baby" breaths.

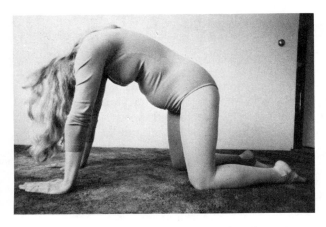

Figure 7C.11 The Cat with an arched back.

Position 8: Leg Stretches in a Cat Position

1. With your back flat and your head in a middle position, shift your weight onto your left leg.
2. Begin to raise the right leg with the knee *bent* as high up in the air as is comfortable. Place your right heel as close to your buttocks as you can. (Figure 7C.12) Hold for five to ten seconds, breathing normally.
3. Carefully straighten out the right leg and push back with your heel, moving your toes toward your knee. Hold for five to ten seconds breathing normally. (Figure 7C.13)
4. Keeping your leg straight, move your toes down to the mat, curling them under. Push your heel close to the mat to s-t-r-e-t-c-h all the muscles in your thigh, calf, and ankle area. Hold five to 30 seconds, breathing normally. (Figure 7C.14)

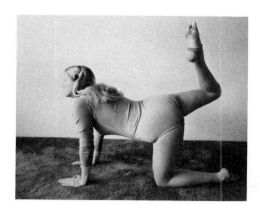

Figure 7C.12 Leg Stretch
with a bent knee.

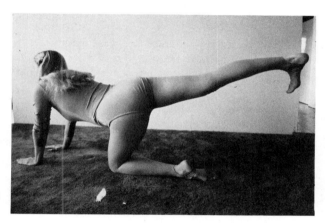

Figure 7C.13 Leg Stretch
with a straight leg.

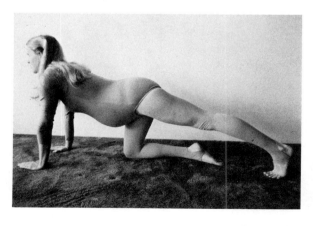

Figure 7C.14 Leg
Stretch with toes curled
under.

5. Bring the outstretched leg back up into the air, bending at the knee and pushing your knee up in the air as high as comfortable. Hold five to ten seconds.

6. Bring the right leg back to the starting position. Then take one to two "Rock-the-Baby" breaths.

7. Repeat these same leg movements on the left side.
   Note: During the last two to three months of your pregnancy, you may want to sit back on your heels in the Zen Sitting Position and take one to five deep breaths before proceeding to the second leg.

Position 9: Arm Stretching in the Zen Sitting Position

1. After completing the second leg stretch, place your buttocks on your heels. If this is uncomfortable, place both feet next to your left hip and proceed.

2. Clasp your hands and raise your arms, palms facing upward, as high above your head as it is comfortable. Stretch the arms and shoulders. Hold for five to ten seconds while breathing normally.

3. Keeping your arms in this position, stretch first to the left, then to the right, without turning. (Figure 7C.15) Hold each position five to ten seconds. Stretch five seconds, pushing your arms back.

4. Lower your hands to your lap and take one to two "Rock-the-Baby" breaths.

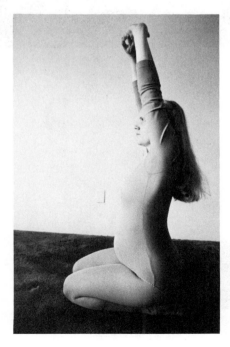

Figure 7C.15   Arm Stretches in the Zen sitting position.

Position 10: Stretching Out of a Squat

1. Placing your hands on the mat beside you, shift into a squatting position with your feet about 12 inches apart and at a 45° angle outward.

2. Put your hands, palms down, on the mat in front of you and take one to four "Baby Breaths." (Figure 7C.16)

3. After the breaths, keep your head up, push on your palms, straighten your legs and raise your buttocks into the air. (Figure 7C.17) *Note:* During the last few weeks of your pregnancy, you may want to use a chair to help you get up.

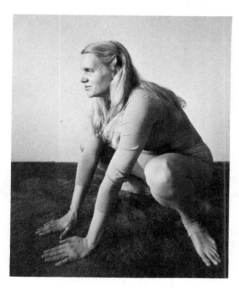

Figure 7C.16 Stretching out of a Squat.

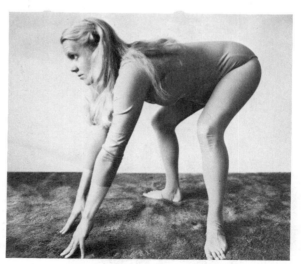

Figure 7C.17 Half way up.

Position 11: Modified Backward Bend

1. When you are balanced, stretch your arms out in front of your chest, palms together; move your arms up toward the ceiling. (Figure 7C.18)
2. Move your arms behind your head and bend slightly backwards. Hold, breathing normally, no more than five seconds. *Note:* If this makes you dizzy or uncomfortable, just stretch upwards rather than backwards.

Figure 7C.18   Modified Backward Bend.

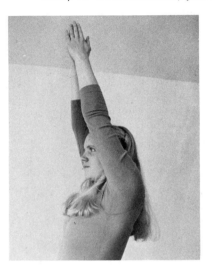

Position 12: Standing Prayer Pose

1. Keeping the palms together, bring them back to your breastbone. (Figure 7C.19)

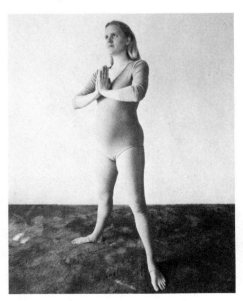

Figure 7C.19   Standing Prayer Position.

2. Take one to two "Rock-the-Baby" breaths and repeat this series one to three times. Follow with a Complete Relaxation (pp. 155–57) for 10–20 minutes.

Cautions and Comments:

- Do not be alarmed at the number of different movements which are contained in this series. Once you have memorized them, you will grow to have your favorite positions. Do not leave out the movements that you do not like. Each movement in this series is beautifully utilitarian for pregnant women.

- Sometimes in the early and later months of your pregnancy, you may experience some dizziness coming up out of the squat (#10). If this happens, shift onto your knees in a kneeling position with the rest of the body straight and proceed with the described arm movements.

- As you practice this series, try to increase the number of seconds you hold each position. You should never exceed 30 seconds in any one position.

- Try to include one "Salute to the Child" series in all your practice sessions.

- A practice cassette tape is available for Salute to the Child. See Appendix for further details.

D: STANDING ASANAS

Your legs may tire and swell more easily during pregnancy; the following postures may be very helpful for invigorating them. Remember to practice a variety of postures during each practice session. Choose one or two of the following postures to add to your daily routine. Try each posture at least once to get the feeling of it.

Pregnancy Triangle

Benefits:

- Relieves backache while stretching and strengthening the spine
- Tones the hip, thigh, buttocks, and leg muscles
- Keeps part of your waistline intact (every little bit helps!)
- Keeps your shoulders limber

Directions:

1. Stand with your feet as wide apart as comfortable.

2. Turn your right foot at a 45° angle while keeping the left foot facing forward.

3. Stretch both arms out to your sides palms down. (Figure 7D.1)

4. Bend the right knee and stretch the right arm down toward the floor.

5. Place the right hand on the floor next to your right foot or on your right ankle.

6. Place your left arm next to your left ear and stretch the left arm forward.

7. Hold five to ten seconds or as long as is comfortable, breathing normally. (Figure 7D.2)

8. Return to starting position with arms outstretched. Exhale arms down and then take two to three ''Rock-the-Baby'' breaths.

9. Repeat movements on your left side.

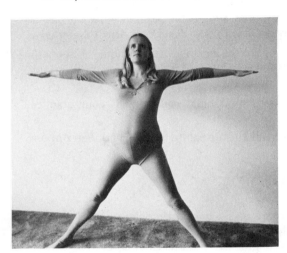

Figure 7D.1   Preparation for the Triangle.

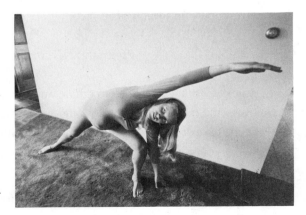

Figure 7D.2   The Pregnancy Triangle.

Cautions and Comments:
- During the later months, you may want to have a chair next to you to help you get back up.
- You can maximize the stretch to your waist by stretching the top arm further forward.
- Don't let the top arm droop toward the floor; always keep it parallel to the floor and stretched.

Side Lunge

This should be practiced in a standing position.

Benefits:
- Tones, firms, and stretches the inner thighs, legs, buttocks, and arms
- Helps to strengthen and stretch the birth canal area (pelvic floor muscles)
- Reduces tension and stiffness in arms, neck, and back

Directions: Variation I:
1. Standing straight with your legs as wide open as is comfortable, turn your right foot out 90° to the side.
2. Bending your right leg, shift your weight to your right leg and lunge over to the right side. (Figure 7D.3) Keep your left leg straight, tightening your knee.

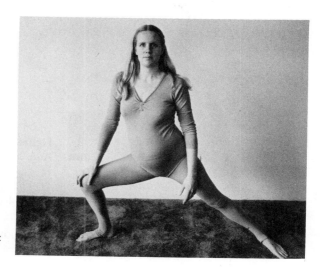

Figure 7D.3 Side Lunge: Variation I.

3. Hold for five to 30 seconds; breathe normally.

4. Return to starting position. Take one to three "Rock-the-Baby" breaths. Repeat on other side.

5. Practice two to three stretches on each side.

Variation II:

1. After you have assumed a lunge position as described in #1–3 above, turn at the waist towards the right side.

2. Stretch your arms out to the sides and then place your palms together above your head as you inhale.

3. Stretch the arms up as you look at your hands and breathe normally. Maximize your stretch and hold for five to 30 seconds. (Figure 7D.4)

4. Exhale as you release the arms and return to starting position.

5. Take two to three "Rock-the-Baby" breaths and repeat on other side.

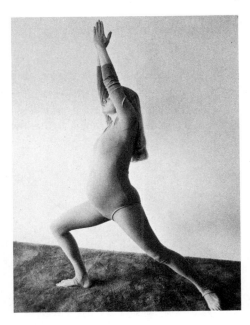

Figure 7D.4 Side Lunge with Arm Stretch: Variation II.

Cautions and Comments:

• Do try to keep the outstretched leg straight and that foot flat on the floor.

• In Variation II, move your arms in back of head to maximize the stretch to your lower back.

E: STANDING ASANAS WITH A CHAIR

Often when you are pregnant, you may feel the urge to really stretch the lower back and spine. Since you cannot practice any postures lying flat on your abdomen, standing postures are a very useful substitute. Do not limit yourself to a chair for practice. The side of the sink during dishwashing breaks will work just as well. Try to find other creative places to practice these stretches. These tension releasing movements work well at 2:00 A.M., when you just cannot seem to get back to sleep.

Half Bow with Chair

This should always be practiced with a chair for support.

Benefits:
- Gives a stimulating stretch to the lower back, thereby releasing tension
- Tones and tightens the thighs, hips, and buttocks
- Helps to prevent groin spasms (round ligament spasms)
- Strengthens the shoulders and arms
- Is helpful for eliminating middle-of-the-night insomnia

Directions:
1. Stand up tall 12 inches behind a chair. Place your right hand on top of the chair.
2. Shift your weight to your right leg keeping it straight, but not locked.
3. Bend your left leg up and place your left hand on the top part of your left foot.
4. Keep your left arm straight as you pull the left leg up and open it as wide as you can. (Figure 7E.1)

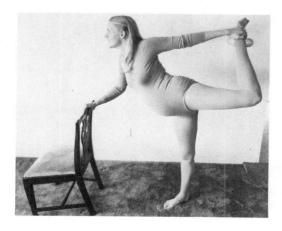

Figure 7E.1   Half Bow with chair.

113

5. Breathe normally as you hold this posture for five to 30 seconds.

6. Lower the left knee down and then release your left foot.

7. With both feet on the ground take two to three "Rock-the-Baby" breaths.

8. Repeat on other side.

Cautions and Comments:
- Bending the arm which you have on the chair will give you better balance.
- You can turn your head and look back at your raised foot for an added stretch to the neck area.
- This is a tension releasing posture which can be used as a quick energizer.
- This can easily be done near your sink if your lower back begins to ache as you do the dishes.
- You can do this stretch with your leg outstretched and both hands on top of the chair. But you should hold the leg lift only five to 30 seconds on each side.

F: POSES IN A FLAT BACK POSITION

During the later months of pregnancy, you may find that lying prone on your back with the full weight of the uterus and baby pressing down on your circulatory system will be very uncomfortable. Some women experience numbness in the legs if they are forced to remain in this position for extended periods of time. The following asanas can be practiced during most of the pregnant months, but they should *never* be done consecutively. You can easily intersperse these postures with side-lying or sitting exercises.

Pendulum Legs

Benefits:
- Massages and releases tension from the lower back
- Relieves lower backache
- Helps to tone the thighs, waist, and buttocks
- Is a very soothing exercise which brings relaxation to the entire body

Directions:
1. Lying on your back, stretch your arms straight out from your shoulders.
2. Bend both legs at the knees and put your legs together and your feet flat on the floor as close to your body as is comfortable. (Figure 7F.1)

3. Begin moving the knees from side to side like a pendulum.

4. Let the knees eventually fall on one side for five to ten seconds. (Figure 7F.2) Repeat on other side.

Figure 7F.1 Preparatory position for Pendulum Legs.

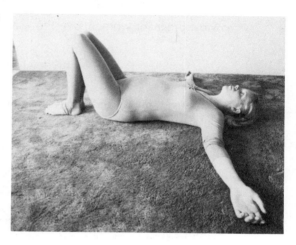

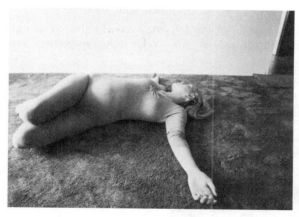

Figure 7F.2 Pendulum Legs with knees on floor.

5. Keep moving the knees in a pendulum motion from side to side until your lower back begins to feel warm and relaxed.

6. Shift into a side-lying position and take two to threee "Rock-the-Baby" breaths.

Cautions and Comments:
- Do this asana only if it feels good.
- Be sure to practice this asana only on a well padded mat. An extra pillow under your lower back is helpful.

- You do not have to keep your feet on the ground as you move your knees from side to side.
- Keep your eyes closed and concentrate on the area of your back which is being massaged.
- Most pregnant women love this asana.

Universal Pose

Benefits:
- Loosens, relaxes, and tones the lower back, which can often ache during pregnancy
- Strengthens the spine while keeping it supple
- Tones the legs, thighs, and buttocks
- Relieves lower backache

Directions:
1. Lying on your back, bend your right leg and place your right foot next to your inside left knee. (Figure 7F.3)
2. Shift your arms so that they extend out from your shoulders.
3. Let your left leg bend slightly at the left knee as you shift your right knee down onto the mat on the left side. Your right hip will roll into the air.
4. Turn your head and look in the opposite direction of your knee. (Figure 7F.4) Try to keep your arms and shoulders as close to the mat as you can comfortably.

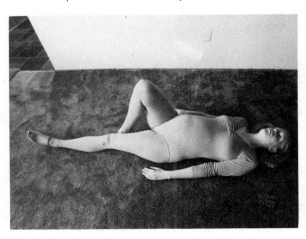

Figure 7F.3 Preparation for the Universal Pose.

Figure 7F.4 The Universal Pose.

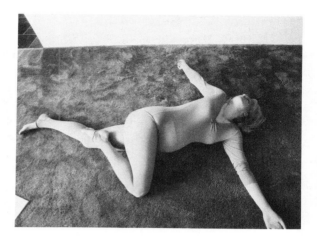

5. Hold this posture five to 30 seconds as you consciously relax your shoulders, hips, and legs. Breathe normally throughout.

6. Return to a starting position leaving the arms outstretched.

7. Take two to three "Rock-the-Baby" breaths and repeat movements on the other side. Repeat this posture twice.

Cautions and Comments:

- You may hear the bones in your back crack as you practice this asana. Do not be alarmed, you are merely breaking up calcium deposits as well as releasing bodily tension and tiredness.

- You may find that bending the leg which is on the bottom a bit more will increase your enjoyment of this asana.

- If the top leg does not want to go down to the mat, you can stretch it down with the closest hand, but do not force it.

The Simple Fish Position

Benefits:

- Relieves tension while limbering the upper back and neck
- Improves circulation to the head
- Is an energizing posture
- Helps to drain excess mucous from the sinuses
- Gives the spine a dynamic backward bend

Directions:

1. Lie on your back with your arms at your sides and your legs straight.

2. Slide your hands, palms down, under your buttocks, elbows slightly out to the side.

3. Half sit up as you push down on your elbows and arch your chest up.

4. Drop your head back and under so that you are resting on the very top of your head. Arch your chest up as high as you can. (Figure 7F.5)

5. Adjust your elbows out to the side for greater comfort. Shift your weight to your buttocks while you relax the legs and feet.

6. Hold for five to 30 seconds or as long as is comfortable while breathing normally.

7. Slowly come out of the asana by flattening down and relaxing in a side lying position. Take two to three "Rock-the-Baby" breaths. Repeat once again.

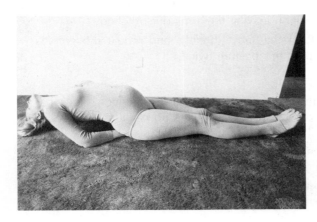

Figure 7F.5 The Simple Fish.

Cautions and Comments:

- Do not breathe too deeply or you may become dizzy.

- This is one of the few backward-bending asanas which is beneficial and *safe* for the pregnant yoga student.

- If you have a cold, this position is quite helpful, for your sinus cavities will drain mucous into your throat so that you can easily spit it out once you have finished practicing.

- This is an excellent posture for women who work in an office and bend forward much of the time because of the counterbalancing stretch.
- This posture will eliminate backaches caused by bad posture, tension, and tiredness.

Flat back postures in the "Basic Nine" series are: Pelvic Rocking (p. 86), the Bridge (pp. 86–89), the Half Sit-Up (pp. 91–92), and the Lower Back Rocker (p. 89). Remember *never* to practice two flat back positions in a row.

G: POSTURES IN A SITTING POSITION

The bigger you grow, the more difficult it becomes to sit in any one position for a long period of time. A variety of sitting positions have already been described and illustrated in the Salute to the Child exercise. In addition, there are a number of other positions which can be most helpful when you feel like a beached whale and cannot seem to find a comfortable way to sit. If you become familiar with and use these sitting positions from the early months of your pregnancy, you should experience more comfort as you grow. Sitting cross-legged is excellent for strengthening your thigh and perineal muscles in preparation for childbirth. However, if you have a varicose vein problem, cross-legged sitting is *not* advised. Use the "Zen Sitting Position" (p. 93) and the "Butterfly" (p. 102) instead. Try to use the following suggestions to increase your physical comfort while sitting during pregnancy:

- When sitting in a chair, bend one leg at the knee and place the foot of the bent leg on the chair next to the other thigh; after a while shift legs so other leg is bent.
- If you are sitting for long periods of time, put your legs up on another chair or an ottoman.
- Change sitting positions often.
- Sit cross-legged on the floor as often as possible during your leisure time. Try it on the sofa. If you have varicose veins use the Zen Sitting Position.
- Be sure your back is supported when you are sitting for long periods of time.

When you are not able to sit in yoga sitting positions and must use conventional sitting apparatus, chairs, sofas, etc., you should pay more attention to your sitting posture. As the center of the body balloons out, there is a tendency for your head to droop forward and for you to develop the "pregnancy slouch." This dreaded postural condition can only lead to one thing: BACKACHE!

Look at Figures 7G.1 and 7G.2

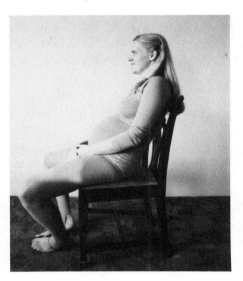

Figure 7G.1 Poor sitting posture.

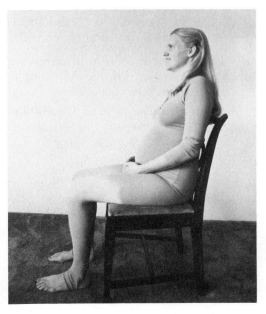

Figure 7G.2 Good sitting posture.

Pregnancy Slouch:
• tummy pushed forward
• lower back unsupported
• shoulders hunched forward
• legs dangling out to the sides

Result:
Pregnancy backache

Good Pregnancy Posture:
• back supported against chair
• tummy weight carried by buttocks and flat feet
• shoulders back and chest forward—mid-back supported by chair

Result:
Vim, vigor and vitality

When you are not sitting on a chair or sofa, you may want to use a Seiza Bench. (See building directions on p. 122.) This Japanese bench was invented to enable people to sit for long periods of meditation. During the last trimester, when any comfortable position is just a fading memory, this bench can become your favorite sitting place.

Sitting on a Seiza Bench

Benefits:
• This marvelous bench will force your spine into correct alignment which will cause your back to feel wonderful
• Ideal for women with varicose veins
• Releases tension from the neck and shoulders
• Increases flexibility in your knees and legs
• Enables you to find a comfortable position for meditation periods

Directions:
1. Resting on your knees, place both feet together. Place the Seiza bench over your lower legs and feet.
2. Lower your bottom onto the bench and sit up straight. (Figure 7G.3)
3. Sit for meditation or to watch television, etc.

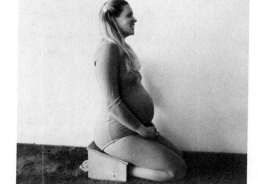

Figure 7G.3 Sitting on a Seiza Bench.

Cautions and Comments:

• You can put a cushion on the top of the bench for more comfort.

• You can read in this position using a coffee table for a book rest.

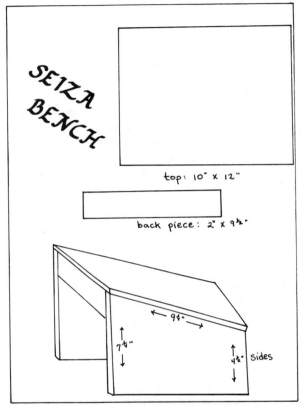

Figure 7G.4 Directions for building a Seiza Bench.

Cross-Legged Sitting Positions

Benefits:

• Improves circulation in your legs

• Strengthens the muscles of the thighs, legs, and spine

• Increases flexibility of the ankles, knees, and hip joints

• Improves your posture

Directions: Simple Cross-Legged Sitting

1. Sit with your knees bent out to the side, ankles crossed in a simple cross-legged position. Place your hands on your knees.

2. Check to see that your spine is straight. If your back is aching, use a wall for support.

3. Remain in this position for as long as is comfortable.

Directions: Half Lotus Position

1. Sit up tall with both legs stretching forward.

2. Bend the left leg and place the left heel as close to the right thigh and the birth canal as possible.

3. Take the right foot in both hands and place it on your left thigh so that the right foot is resting on the crevice created between your left thigh and calf. (Figure 7G.5)

4. Place your hands on your knees and practice your breathing, watch television, read, etc.

5. Hold each side from 30 seconds to five minutes; then change to the other side.

6. When finishing this pose, stretch your legs forward and vibrate your knees.

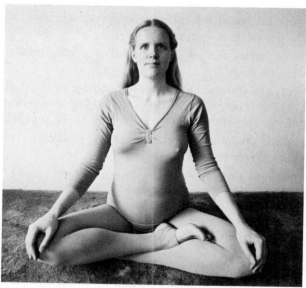

Figure 7G.5   Half Lotus sitting position.

Cautions and Comments:

• If you have a varicose vein condition, all cross-legged sitting positions should be discontinued. Use a Seiza bench, the Zen Sitting Position, or sit in a chair with your feet up.

- If you are comfortable using a cross-legged sitting position, try it on a wide chair while eating dinner.
- Sitting cross-legged will help to strengthen your spine and take some pressure off your lower back.
- Use a cushion under your buttocks if the floor is too hard.

Alternate Leg Stretch to the Side

Benefits:
- Strenghtens and firms the abdomen and the legs
- Relieves and reduces tension from the back, legs, and buttocks
- The abdominal organs are massaged and stimulated into action for better digestion and elimination.
- Energizes the body by making the spine strong and flexible

Directions:
1. Sit on your mat with a straight back in the open "V" leg position. Take one to two "Rock-the-Baby" breaths.
2. Bend your left leg at the knee bringing your left heel as close to the birth canal area as is comfortable.
3. Clasp your hands and inhale while bringing your hands above your head. (Figure 7G.6)
4. Breathing normally and keeping your head between your upper arms, stretch as far down toward the extended leg as is comfortable. Do not hold your breath or bounce. Hold five to 30 sec. (7G.7)
5. Stretch back up into an upright position. Exhale as you lower the hands back down to your knees.
6. Take two to three "Rock-the-Baby" breaths and then repeat movements on the other side.

Cautions and Comments:
- During the early months of your pregnancy, you may find it quite easy to lower your head quite close to your knee. As the baby grows, you may find it uncomfortable to stretch down quite so far. You can hold a towel looped around your foot for increased stretch.
- This asana is highly beneficial for eliminating middle and lower back pain.
- This asana can also be practiced with the legs in an open "V" position with one hand extended and touching the toes or calf of the same leg, and the other hand stretched above and parallel to it (Figure 7G.8).

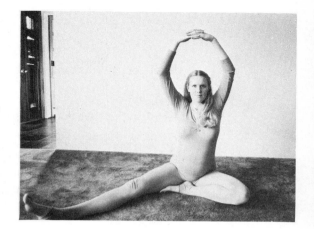

Figure 7G.6 Preparation for Alternate Leg Stretch to the side.

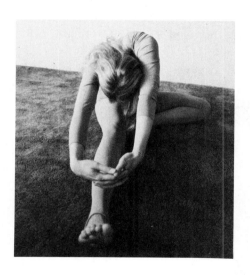

Figure 7G.7 Completed Alternate Leg Stretch to the side.

Figure 7G.8 Alternate Leg Stretch in Open "V" position.

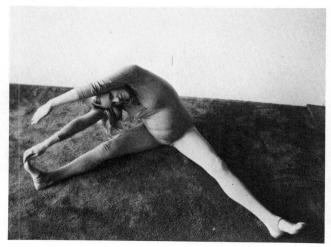

Cow Head Pose

This can be practiced sitting or standing.

Benefits:
- Helps to improve rounded shoulders and poor posture
- Helps to counterbalance the extra weight of your breasts
- Strengthens and firms your upper arms
- Releases tension in the shoulders while exercising the muscles near your shoulder blades and in the upper back

Directions:
1. Sit straight in any comfortable position.
2. Bend your left arm and bring it behind your back with your palm facing out. Try to move it as far up your back as you can.
3. Bring your right arm straight up and bend it trying to bring it to the center of your back.
4. Try to bring the hands as close together as you can and eventually interlock the hands. (Figure 7G.9)
5. Keep the top elbow straight up in the air. (This is called the Cow Head Pose because the upper elbow is supposed to look like a cow's horn.)

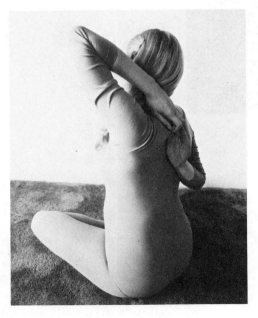

Figure 7G.9 The Cow Head Pose.

6. Hold for five to 30 seconds, or as long as comfortable, as you gently pull upward with the right hand, then downward with the left hand. Breathe normally throughout.

7. Separate the hands and repeat on the other side. Repeat twice.

Cautions and Comments:

• Do not be dismayed if you cannot clasp your hands. Simply hold a small towel or handkerchief in the top hand and clasp it with the bottom hand and stretch. Eventually the hands will clasp.

• If you are right-handed, you will probably find that the left side is very difficult to clasp. The opposite is true for left-handed people.

• This is an excellent exercise for pregnant women who are working at a desk. It will reduce accumulated tension in the shoulders.

• Remember to keep your back straight throughout this asana.

Pose of the Moon

Benefits:

• Improves flexibility in the legs and knees

• Releases tension in the shoulders and arms

• Gently stretches and strengthens the spine and back muscles

• Is a quick energizer

Directions:

1. Sit in the Zen Sitting position by bending both legs and sitting on your heels. Separate your knees six to eight inches apart.

2. Sit up straight, raise both arms. Stretch as high above your head as possible.

3. Hold the stretch as you move the arms down to the floor in front of you. Place your forehead on the mat. (Figure 7G.10)

Figure 7G.10 The completed Moon Pose.

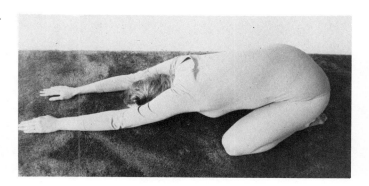

4. Stretch your arms and fingers as far in front of you as is comfortable. Breathe normally as you hold for ten to 60 seconds.

5. Stretch the arms back up into the air and then float them down to your sides as you exhale.

6. Repeat twice.

Cautions and Comments:
- As the pregnancy progresses, you may want to have a pillow on the floor for your head.
- When the uterus is expanded to its highest height, usually during the eighth and ninth months, you may find this asana uncomfortable.
- This posture can easily be done at your desk if you are working in an office. It is very effective as an energizer and tension releaser.

Elbow Circles

This can be practiced in any comfortable upright position.

Benefits:
- Loosens, relaxes, and releases tension from the shoulders and lower neck areas
- Helps to prevent headaches

Directions:
1. Bend your arms and place the palms of your hands on your shoulders with your fingers facing in toward your neck.
2. Begin to make circles with your elbows. (Figure 7G.11)

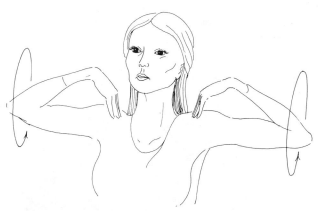

Figure 7G.11 Elbow Circles.

3. Make five very large circles forward and then reverse and make five circles backward.

4. Bring your hands back into your lap and take one to two "Rock-the-Baby" breaths.

Cautions and Comments:

• This posture is highly recommended for women who work at desks or on any job which requires forward bending. Use it often during your work day.

• An interesting variation can be experienced by pushing the elbows as far behind you as you can, keeping your hands on your shoulders. Hold for a count of five and then move the elbows in front of you. Hold again for a count of five as you touch your elbows together. Release and breathe.

• You may hear cracking in the shoulder area as you practice this pose. This is a sign of tightness in this area, which you are breaking up.

H: EXERCISES FOR THE PELVIC FLOOR OR BIRTH CANAL MUSCLES

Prior to pregnancy the muscles of the pelvic floor are used for elimination and sexual purposes. With the advent of the growing uterus and impending birth, these muscles become much more significant. You may have gone through your life until this time not really being aware that you have a layer of muscles which form a sling or support system across the bottom of your pelvis. The easiest way to familiarize yourself with these muscles is to do the following exercises: (Figure 7H.1)

Pelvic Floor Exercise (or Sexercises)

Benefits:

• Strengthens the pelvic floor, thereby giving better support to your uterus

• Prevents trickling urine while sneezing, laughing, coughing, etc.

• Helps to prevent damage to the birth canal during the birth of the child

• Helps to relieve pelvic congestion or swelling during pregnancy

• Helps prevent or alleviate hemorrhoids.

Directions:

1. Next time you go into the bathroom to urinate, stop your urine flow after only half of the water is passed.

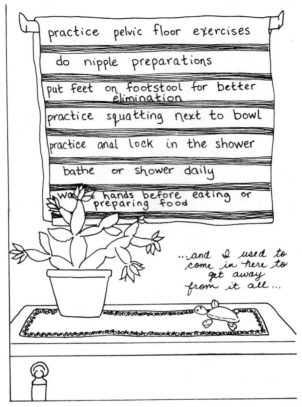

On the shade:

practice pelvic floor exercises

do nipple preparations

put feet on footstool for better elimination

practice squatting next to bowl

practice anal lock in the shower

bathe or shower daily

wash hands before eating or preparing food

...and I used to come in here to get away from it all...

Figure 7H.1

2. Close your eyes and feel the contracted pelvic floor muscles.

3. Void a bit more and then contract again.

4. Contract your pelvic floor muscles four to five times each time you urinate until you are totally familiar with these muscles.

5. Once you know how to contract these muscles, do this exercise when you are not urinating several times a day. Hold each contraction for two seconds working up to 300 contractions a day. It sounds like a lot of work, but it really takes very little time.

Cautions and Comments:
- Many people call these exercises either Kegel's (for the doctor who first made them popular) or sexercises. Once you strengthen and tone the pelvic floor, you will find your sexual pleasure will increase. Your partner can check your tone while you are making love. The tighter the muscles, the higher the pleasure quotient, so keep practicing . . .

- Make a mental note to do these exercises at red lights, during commercials, in the bathroom, etc.

The Anal Lock

See Part B of this chapter, the "Basic Nine," Posture 7, for full details.

The Elevator

Benefits:
- Strengthens the muscles which will be utilized during childbirth
- Exercises all the inner muscles of the pelvic floor
- Helps to keep the sexual area alive and responsive

Directions:
1. In any comfortable position, focus your awareness on your vaginal or birth canal area muscles. Take one "Rock-the-Baby" breath and exhale.
2. Imagine that your pelvic floor muscles are an elevator which is slowly moving from the first to the sixth floor. Slowly begin to pull your muscles up toward your spine. You may feel a slight tightening in the lowest part of the abdomen.
3. Really concentrate and feel the muscles on the first floor, second floor, etc. Hold the elevator at the sixth floor for five to ten seconds and then slowly lower.
4. Control the descent to the first floor and then lower to the basement by pushing down.
5. Repeat the trip two to three times, then relax, taking two to three "Rock-the-Baby" breaths.

Cautions and Comments:
- As your muscle tone increases, it will become much easier to hold the elevator on the top floor.
- After you deliver the elevator to the basement, relax all the muscles of the pelvic floor completely to learn that sensation. You will have to relax this area at will during delivery to facilitate the birth of your child.

Baby Breath

See Chapter 2 for complete details.

MAKING LOVE DURING PREGNANCY

The preceding exercises will focus your attention on, as well as tone and strengthen, your sexual muscles. They may also heighten your sexual desires during pregnancy. Sharing your feelings about your sexuality with your mate, either verbally or via a letter, is very important for your well being. Commonly women experience a decrease in sexual desire during the first trimester, increased interest and pleasure during the second trimester and a decrease, due to size, during the third trimester. Keeping your husband informed about your changing desires and reactions can eliminate many problems and frustrations. Ask your mate his views about the desirability of your pregnant body. This exchange of ideas and opinions can have a very definite effect on your sex life while you are pregnant. New ideas and reactions will be crossing both of your minds. Many men have underlying fears of hurting the baby while making love. Many women feel the need for more closeness via hugging or massage rather than having intercourse. Each couple's reactions are uniquely their own and should be explored for a more positive pregnancy experience. Having both partners read and discuss the book, *Making Love During Pregnancy,* by Elisabeth Bing and Libby Colman (Bantam Books, 1977) can help them explore new horizons. This honest and open book contains beautiful illustrations and direct quotes from many couples about their sexual experiences.

You may wonder how yoga has a connection to sexual activity, since many people equate strict yoga practice with celibacy. The aspect of yoga which has been developed within this book is especially for people in the mainstream of life, rather than those who have limited their activities. The goal of yoga practice is physical, mental, and spiritual development, and sexual relations can play a very vital part in this development.

Since pregnancy affords you freedom from birth control techniques, there can be more spontaneity in your sexual pursuits. The challenge of an ever enlarging female body can lead to more creative lovemaking. The combination of these two factors can add new dimensions to the sexual aspect of your lives. If you have been practicing your asanas on a regular basis, you will find that you have become more flexible, and thereby capable, of holding positions for longer periods of time. Another aspect of pregnancy is heightened sensitivity.

The same inner energy which is responsible for your emotional ups and downs can be used quite pleasurably during lovemaking. This inner energy often increases your physical bodily responses, thereby enabling you to reach and feel deeper sexual pleasure. These responses can be used even if you are not making love. A mutual massage (see Chapter 11 for full details) can be extremely enjoyable and satisfying for both partners, if lovemaking is not feasible or desired. It is another aspect of being close and giving pleasure to one another.

Pregnancy may be the first time a couple will explore other ways of pleasuring each other. Developing new ways during the middle pregnancy months may prove quite helpful during the time just before and right after your baby is born. Many women have indicated feelings of pride or increased femininity when they learned to bring their mates to orgasm in a new way. Other women were relieved to know that a heightened sexual drive could be relieved by masturbation without any ill effects on the baby. Many couples discover mutual masturbation during the waiting months. These preparatory months are definitely the right time to explore and deepen your physical bodily experiences.

One very opportune time to find out the strength of your birth canal (pelvic floor) muscles is during lovemaking. Simply contract your pelvic floor muscles and ask your mate about the tightness of the contraction. This can lead to a lot of laughing (as reported by some of my students) but increased practicing. One husband used to suggest practicing the sexercises *every time* he wanted to make love. His wife reported that he thought this gave the lovemaking a very noble and worthwhile reason!

Another yogic technique which may increase or prolong your sexual pleasure is simultaneous breathing once both partners have reached orgasm. This breathing doesn't have to be deep, just mutual. Try to breathe in unison as you hold the embrace. Concentrate on the physical union which you are experiencing.

A variety of new physical positions is open to you at this time as well. As the abdomen grows larger, it may be advisable for the woman to be on top. You may find the use of chair with an ottoman next to it quite helpful. Your husband can lie on the chair and ottoman with you above him with your feet on the floor and hands on the ottoman. In this position, you can guide the depth of penetration as well as the rhythm of movement. This position can be adapted for the corner of the bed, again with the woman's feet on the floor (if the woman is not too tall). Other couples have indicated that rear entry positions with the woman either lying down or standing are helpful as well. The key word at this time is *experiment*. Try out a variety of positions and find the ones you like best.

Many women report that having followed the advice to experiment, they find themselves spending a great deal of time laughing at some of the results. Laughter and joking can add the light touch which is needed, especially during the last weeks of pregnancy. Some of your experiments may end with making jokes rather than making love, while others may be very satisfying. By keeping this area of your life as positive and light-hearted as possible, you will strengthen your marriage and come to realize new facets of the love you share.

I: LEG STRETCHES USING A WALL

Using a combination of gravity and imagination, you can quickly lighten and revitalize aching legs. The combination of added body weight and body volume often creates leg problems during pregnancy. By simply putting your feet up and retiring from the world for a few moments each day, you can minimize this problem while you increase your vitality and productivity. You should find the following wall stretches quite enjoyable and useful, even if you are not experiencing any leg problems during your pregnancy. Since inverted postures are not highly recommended during pregnancy, these wall stretches are a fine substitute.

45° Leg Rester

This can only be practiced lying on your back.

Benefits:
- Drains the legs of excess blood via gravity
- Relieves tired and swollen feet, ankles, and legs
- Rests the large blood vessels and valves within the legs
- Helps to prevent or aid varicose veins

Directions:
1. Lying flat on the floor, place your legs at a 45° angle against a wall. (Figure 71.1)

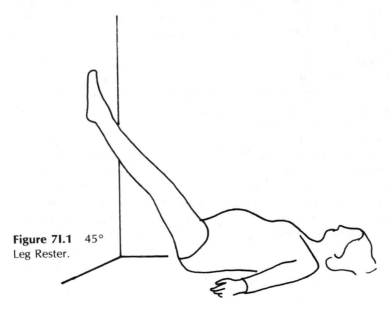

Figure 71.1 45°
Leg Rester.

2. Place your hands several inches from your body, palms up or down and center your head.

3. Close your eyes and imagine your legs are bathing in a cool pool of water. Imagine the lovely scenery near the pool. See the blue sky, the variety of trees, the colorful flowers, hear the singing of the birds. Paint your mental scene as fully as you can. Leave out any disturbances such as mosquitoes, bugs, loud noises, etc. You can choose a mountain scene during one practice session and a tropical scene during another. Try to make the scene as real as you can. Imagine yourself in this wonderful magical scene.

4. Feel the cool water washing away the tiredness and tension from your legs and feet.

5. Breathe rhythmically and smoothly as you embellish your beautiful private pool.

6. Remain in this position up to a maximum of five minutes.

7. Slowly rouse yourself by moving your fingers first, then your toes. Take a deep breath and let it go as you begin to stretch.

8. Bend your knees and bring them down on one side of you. Roll over to that side and slowly, using your hands, walk yourself up into a sitting position.

Cautions and Comments:
- Do not remain in this position long enough to feel your legs numb or going to sleep. Hold only as long as the legs feel comfortable.
- You can practice a Complete Relaxation (p. 96) in this position as well.
- Doing ten rounds of Alternate Nostril Breathing (pp. 16–18) may be helpful too.

Open "V," Butterfly, and Squat Positions on the Wall

Benefits:
- Stretches the birth canal area open to its fullest, thereby preparing it for childbirth
- Relieves varicose veins by draining the excess blood out of your legs
- Relaxes the veins and valves in the legs
- Relieves tired and swollen feet, ankles and legs
- Stretches and tones the inner thighs

Directions for Open "V":

1. Slide your buttocks up against the wall with the legs extended straight up.
2. Let your legs open and slide down into an open "V" position. (Figure 71.2)
3. Keep your knees loose and do not point your toes.
4. Hold one to three minutes, breathing normally and consciously relaxing the tight muscles in your legs and groin area. Go back to your imaginary pool to relax and revitalize your legs.
5. Slowly rouse and bring the legs back to the center, push away from the wall, bend the knees, and bring them down on one side. Roll over to that side and, using your hands, walk yourself up into a sitting position.
6. Take one to two "Rock-the-Baby" breaths.

Directions for Butterfly and Wall Squat:

1. Slide your buttocks up against the wall with the legs extended straight up.
2. Bend your knees and bring the soles of your feet together. Let your knees hang out to the side as the backs of your legs lean against the wall in a Butterfly position. (Figure 71.3)
3. Or go into a wall squat by bending your knees on either side of the baby and placing your feet flat against the wall. (Figure 71.4)
4. Breathe normally and evenly in either position holding for 30 seconds to three minutes. Keep your mental concentration on the stretching of the birth canal area. Become familiar with this open feeling. Go back to your private pool and have a dip to cool and refresh your legs.
5. Straighten up your legs and bring them back to the center. Come down following direction #5.
6. Take one to two "Rock-the-Baby" breaths.

Cautions and Comments:

- Some women find these positions uncomfortable. If you are in this category, do not practice them.
- You can build up to two to three minutes in either of these positions if you like.
- Check to see that the rest of your body is relaxed, especially your facial muscles, while you are practicing the open "V," Butterfly, or Squatting on the Wall.

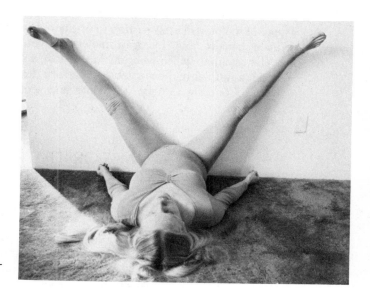

Figure 71.2 Open "V" Position on the wall.

Figure 71.3 The Butterfly on the wall.

Figure 71.4 Squatting on the wall.

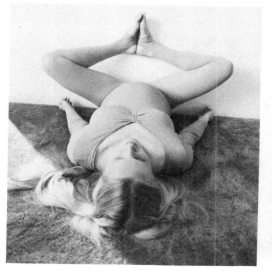

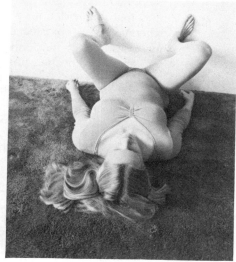

137

As soon as you begin to notice some swelling in your ankles, choose any of the poses in this section to practice. If your swelling continues, immediately speak to your doctor or midwife for you may be experiencing excessive water retention which warrants further care and advice. Some water retention is quite normal and acceptable, especially during the last six weeks of pregnancy. Continue to keep your fluid and protein intake high and your diet balanced.

J: ASANAS FOR THE EXPERIENCED YOGA PRACTITIONER

You may be wondering how you can qualify as an "Experienced Yoga Practitioner."

You must have practiced physical (hatha) yoga for at least a year. This would include taking classes or studying on your own via books. It is important to be honest with yourself about your past practice because some of the asanas contained in this section can cause you some problems if you have not had this previous training and practice. The more advanced postures contained herein have been revised to accommodate the pregnant body. During the earlier months of your pregnancy, you may want to practice the Shoulder Stand and Plough in the normal manner. But as your waist disappears and your weight centers change, adjustments have to be made. Safety should be foremost in your mind while you are practicing. Using a chair for support may have been a sign of weakness or only for "old" people before your pregnancy, but now the situation is very different. Also you may find that you will not be able to hold a posture for as long as you did when you were not pregnant. Always keep in mind that your blood volume increases up to 50% during pregnancy. This is exceedingly important when you are in an inverted posture such as the Shoulder Stand. Listen to your body's signals and come out of the posture as soon as it becomes uncomfortable. Be sure to check the "Cautions and Comments" section of each asana before you practice it.

Full Lotus Sitting Position

Benefits:
- Helps the spine to have a good natural curve, thereby improving posture
- Tones the nerves and circulates blood in the abdominal organs
- Creates a perfect tripod on which to balance the body, even if it is pregnant

- Relieves stiffness and tension in the back, knees, and ankles
- Helps to strengthen the muscles used in delivery

Directions:

1. Sit upright with your legs extended.
2. Clasp your right foot and place it as high as you can on the top of the left thigh.
3. Bend your left knee while you clasp your left foot and place the foot as high on the right thigh as you can comfortably.
4. Hold for 30 seconds to several minutes while breathing normally. (Figure 7J.1)
5. Undo your legs and repeat on the other side with your left foot on the top of the right thigh.

Cautions and Comments:

- Make sure that your head, neck, and back are up straight when in this posture.
- Do not force your legs into this position just to say that you can do a Lotus. (This position sometimes becomes a status symbol among

Figure 7J.1 The Lotus Position.

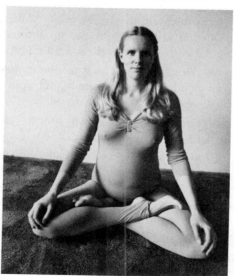

yoga students—pregnant or not!) Never force your knees into this position for you can do damage to the knee area.

- This position, if it is comfortable for you, is excellent for daily meditation or for breathing exercises.
- Your knees may take a while to finally drop down to the floor. Keep trying and eventually, they will.

Pregnancy Shoulder-Stand

Benefits:
- Tones up and soothes the central nervous system
- Helps to relieve aching legs and varicose veins
- Firms and stretches the muscles of the legs, back, neck, and abdomen

Directions:
1. Lie on your back with your buttocks right next to the wall, legs bent, feet flat on wall, hands at your sides, palms down. (Figure 7J.2)
2. Press against the wall to lift the buttocks off the floor. (Figure 7J.3)
3. Bending your arms at the elbows, place your hands on your lower back for support as you straighten the torso and thighs up. (Figure 7J.4)
4. Once you have balanced the baby area on your shoulders and upper back, lift the feet off the wall and find your balance point. (Figure 7J.5)
5. Relax your legs by bending the knees a bit. Make circles with your ankles to loosen that area. Consciously go through all the parts of the body, especially your face, and relax all parts you are not using.
6. Breathe normally. Holding 15 seconds to one minute. When you feel pressure in your head, bend your knees, put your feet back on the wall, and reverse your steps to come down.
7. Once you have come all the way down, shift to the side and assume a side lying or flat back position to rest.
8. Take two to three "Rock-the-Baby" breaths and relax. (Remember to follow the Shoulder-Stand with the Fish.)

Cautions and Comments:
- Use of the wall for going up is imperative since double leg lifts are not recommended during pregnancy.
- If at any time you feel increased pressure in your head, dizziness, or nausea after doing the Shoulder Stand, it should be discontinued.

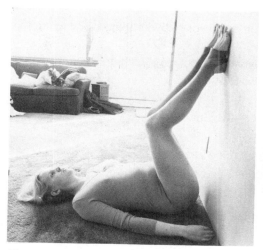

Figure 7J.2 Preparation for a Pregnancy Shoulder Stand.

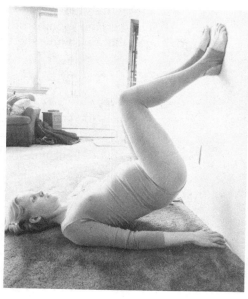

Figure 7J.3 Using the wall to go up.

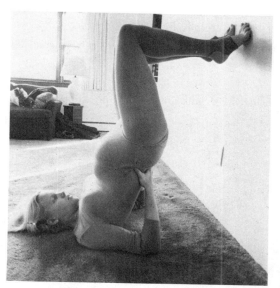

Figure 7J.4 Almost into a Shoulder Stand.

Figure 7J.5 The Pregnancy Shoulder Stand.

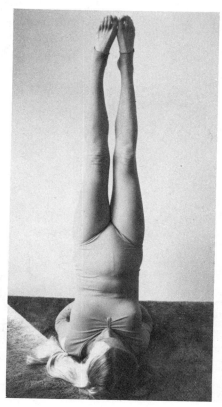

- You should check with your doctor or midwife before practicing this posture on a daily basis.
- In the later months of pregnancy, you may want to keep your feet on the wall during the entire posture.

Pregnancy Advanced Fish

Benefits:
- Limbers the knees, hips, and spine
- Releases tension from the neck and upper back
- Improves circulation to the head while helping to clear the sinuses
- Improves the breathing capacity when the uterus is very high in the chest

Directions:
1. Sit in the Zen Sitting Position (sitting on your heels) and then separate the legs as far as possible.
2. Place your hands right next to your hips, palms down, and *slowly* lower your upper body back putting your weight on your elbows. The elbows will naturally lower to the mat as you lean back.
3. When you are fully leaning on your elbows, separate them a bit, arch the chest, and drop your head carefully back and under.
4. Place the top part of your head on the mat as you arch your spine as high as possible. (Figure 7J.6)

Figure 7J.6 Pregnancy Advanced Fish with a Zen sitting position.

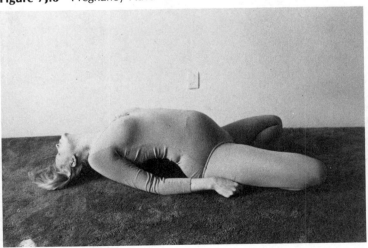

5. Inhale and exhale normally. Deep breathing may cause you to feel nauseated. Hold for five to 30 seconds.

6. Then lower your back and head to the mat. Take one to two "Rock-the-Baby" breaths.

7. Roll over to your left side and, using your hands, push yourself up into a sitting position.

8. Straighten out your legs and vibrate the knees and the legs for several moments.

9. Take two to three "Rock-the-Baby" breaths and relax.

Cautions and Comments:

• Although you may have practiced the Fish posture with no ill effects when you were not pregnant, you may find your body reacting differently during your pregnancy. If you experience negative side effects from this posture, discontinue its practice until after your baby is born.

• This posture can also be practiced with a full Lotus and the hands grasping onto the feet.

The Pregnant Plough

Benefits:

• Relieves lower backache

• Helps to make the spine supple

• Tones the nervous system

• Slims and firms the hips and thighs

Directions:

1. Place a sturdy chair about eight inches behind your head as you assume the same position against the wall which you used for the Shoulder Stand.

2. Follow directions 1–4 for the Shoulder Stand. Once you have found your balance, with your hands on your waist area, lower your feet down to the chair behind you.

3. Stretch your arms away from your hips and clasp the hands. (Figure 7J.7)

4. Hold for five seconds to one minute while breathing normally. Keep your facial muscles loose and check your body for tight areas. Make them relax.

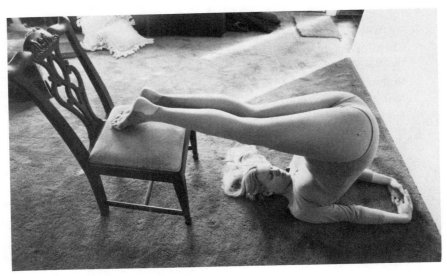

Figure 7J.7   The Pregnant Plough.

5. To come out of this posture, place your hands on your waist and raise the legs up. Bend the legs and place them on the wall. Lower your back and buttocks to the mat.

6. Shift to the side so that you are lying parallel to the wall (watch out for the chair!) and go into a side lying position to rest.

7. Take two to three "Rock-the-Baby" breaths and relax.

Cautions and Comments:

• Practice the pregnant plough as a separate posture from the Shoulder Stand. Although you may have practiced the Shoulder Stand and the Plough together before your pregnancy, it is not advisable to practice them as a series at this time. Remember, if you have pressure in your head, come down immediately.

• Many women find it is difficult to breathe (usually during the seventh through ninth months of pregnancy) while in the Plough position. This Pregnancy Plough variation often helps. However, if you have any difficulty breathing, discontinue the practice of this posture until after the birth of your baby.

• You can open your legs on the chair and stretch your arms under the chair (behind your head) as a variation.

• Remember to keep your knees straight when your legs are back on the chair.

Other advanced asanas to practice are the camel, pose of a child (open your knees), and balancing poses (use a chair).

Do not practice the following asanas: headstand; full forward bending (head to knee) positions; standing backward bends; the wheel; cobra, locust, bow; and the abdominal lift.

The illustrated asanas within this section accentuate the blood flow to your head. If at any time during your pregnancy you should experience head pressure or pressure in your eyes, discontinue practicing these asanas and consult your doctor or midwife. The body has to make many adjustments as your child is growing. It is imperative that you tune into these changes and modify your practices accordingly. A short while after your baby arrives all 84,000 yoga asanas will be available for you to practice!

K: ASANAS AND BREATHING EXERCISES FOR THE WORKING PREGNANT WOMAN

You may have seen some exercises in this book which you would like to practice *if* you had the time. Now that working throughout the pregnant months is more acceptable, increasing numbers of women find themselves in this situation. It is extremely difficult to fit a daily yoga practice session into a schedule that begins early in the morning and ends late in the evening. You may think about practicing yoga and then feel really guilty that you have not done it. Those kinds of thoughts defeat the whole purpose of practicing. With this situation in mind, I have compiled a list of asanas and breathing exercises which you can fit into your working day. By including these movements during your working hours, or your lunch and break time, you will have more energy and feel better by the end of the day. If you do get positive results, you will be much more inclined to practice the pregnancy asanas on the weekend. (Check the appendix for a complete listing of practice cassette tapes which are available for use in conjunction with this book. You may find the tapes will induce you to practice.) The following breaths can be easily practiced while you are working without anyone detecting that you are practicing yoga.

Pranayamas or Breathing Exercises:
- *Rock-the-Baby Breath* (pp. 13–14)
- *Smooth Breath* (10 rounds) (pp. 20–21)

Benefits:
- For calming down and reenergizing
- For centering a harried brain and energizing

- *Sighing Breath* (quietly) (p. 20)

- *Single Nostril Breath* (p. 19) (in the ladies' room is best . . .)

- For releasing tensions when the going gets rough and there isn't even enough time to complain

- When you are falling asleep and it's only 1:30 in the afternoon . . .

Stretching on the Job

It is a good idea to talk with your co-workers about your interest in learning yoga while you are pregnant. Tell them how learning to relax using yogic techniques can help to shorten your laboring time. The reason for these explanations is not my desire to develop a vocal group of yoga admirers (that would be nice . . .), but rather to eliminate the strange looks you may receive if a co-worker walks in on you while you are practicing one of the following asanas.

Daily Reminders
- If you sit a great deal at work, put your feet up on a footstool or a chair to prevent heavy, tired legs

- Walk around once every hour for one or two minutes to keep your body invigorated and improve your circulation

- Keep nutritious snacks handy

Neck, Shoulder and Arm Stretches

These exercises are dearly loved and used by pregnant women who work at desks.

Neck Rolls (pp. 79–81) (Do these three times each way). The exercise eases tension from the neck and shoulders while preventing and/or eliminating headaches.

Cow-Head Pose (pp. 126–27) Do these two times on each side. It eliminates poor posture due to excessive forward bending from typing, office work, factory work, etc.

Chest Expansion (pp. 94–96) Note the office variation of this exercise. Place your arms over the top back of your chair. Interlock your hands and raise them up. This will push your shoulder blades together. Hold five to 30 seconds, breathing normally. Lower the arms and repeat two to three more times. The chest expansion opens the chest area and relieves tired shoulders and arms. This movement is a quick energizer.

Elbow Circles (pp. 128–29) This should be practiced twice a day while working. Five circles forward and five circles backward. It will loosen, relax, and renew the shoulders and upper arms; eliminate tight shoulders and desk stoop; and help prevent headaches.

Pose of the Moon (pp. 128–29) The office variation follows: Sit at a desk or a table, and stretch your arms up toward the ceiling. Stretch them forward placing the palms of your hands on the top of the desk or table. Place your chin or forehead on the desk surface and stretch the arms forward for 10–30 seconds. Return to a starting position. Repeat two times more. Take a breath ("Rock-the-Baby" or "Baby Breath") between stretches and then get back to work. This will release tension from the entire spine, shoulders, and arms. When you feel like giving up, try this pose!

Arm Stretches to the Side (p. 106) This is Salute to the Child, position #9. Sitting at your desk or standing on the job, interlock your hands and stretch them up above your head, palms up. S-t-r-e-t-c-h. Stretch to the right. Hold five seconds. Stretch to the left. Hold five seconds. Return to work. This exercise stretches the upper torso, thereby eliminating tension. It is a quick energizer for the arms, back, and shoulders.

Back Stretches

Sitting Spinal Twist (pp. 85–86) Sitting at your desk or in a chair with a steady back, turn around and place both your hands on the top of the chair. Keep your feet and legs facing forward. Look over your back shoulder and relax all muscles you are not using. Hold five to 30 seconds. Return to center, take one or two "Rock-the-Baby" breaths and relax. Repeat on other side. This exercise strengthens the spine while it simultaneously eliminates tiredness. It also helps to improve your posture.

Foot and Calf Stretches

Foot Circles Sitting at your desk or in a chair, slowly start to rotate your feet at the ankle. Make five circles in one direction. Change directions and do five circles. Then consciously relax the feet: start with the toes and slowly work your way up the foot until the feet feel tingly and light. Foot circles increase circulation to the ankles and feet. They also help eliminate tired aching feet.

Foot Rolls Stand 12 inches behind your chair. Place your hands on top of the back of the chair. Go up on your toes. Hold five seconds.

Shift onto the outsides of your feet. Hold five seconds. Shift onto the heels of your feet (lift rest of foot up) and hold five seconds; shift onto the insides of the feet (go knock-kneed) and hold five seconds. Repeat twice. Your feet should feel cooler and lighter. This increases circulation to the feet and legs, helps to eliminate tired and swollen legs and feet and is an energizing posture.

Calf Stretches Sitting at your desk or in a chair, straighten your legs and raise them about 12–15 inches off the ground. Push your heels forward and point your toes toward your knees. Hold 20–60 seconds and release. Repeat twice. Take one or two ''Rock-the-Baby'' breaths between stretches; then return to looking busy. These stretches help prevent cramping in the calf area, which is so prevalent in pregnancy. They also help keep the legs in good tone.

Part II
Labor and Birth

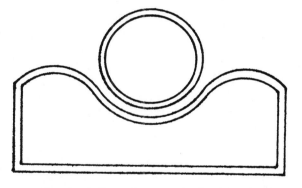

Ancient Egyptian symbol of birth

Eight
Complete Relaxation Self-Taught

The most important skill which must be learned for active participation in the birth process is the ability to relax at will. Most people do not fully understand the training which is necessary to acquire this skill.

In this country, we *do things* to relax. We play tennis, we do needlepoint, we watch television, we read, etc. We usually call these things forms of relaxation. Actually, these things are activities which we enjoy doing, so we think of them as forms of relaxation.

From a yogic point of view, the only effective form of relaxation is a body at rest and consciously relaxed. You may be thinking that this describes what you do every night when you go to sleep. There is one major difference between relaxation and sleep. When you fall off to sleep, you are no longer conscious. When you learn to do a Complete Relaxation, you keep your awareness.

The best and most effective way to learn progressive relaxation is to practice it over and over and over again. It is an acquired skill which takes time, practice, and patience to develop. By continually commanding and allowing the body to relax, you will become totally familiar with this state of being. Once you have mastered this skill, you can use it in a variety of different situations. When you are in active labor, you can consciously enter this state at will between contractions, thereby saving your energy for the coming contraction. This same skill is invaluable if you are nursing your baby. Your physical relaxation will enable your milk to let down and will make the nursing experience more pleasurable and successful for both you and the child.

As you grow larger, you may find it more and more difficult to find comfortable positions. For that reason, a variety of suggested relaxation positions have been included. Try to choose and use only one position when you practice Complete Relaxation. If you give yourself the option of changing positions, you may spend the entire time shifting from one position to another rather than practicing relaxation. Try a Complete Relaxation at least once in all of the following positions to familiarize yourself with how each position feels.

The Sponge Position

Benefits:
- Is a position most people associate with relaxation
- Evenly distributes your body weight

Directions:
1. Lie flat on your back, head centered on the mat with a pillow under your head and upper back for comfort.
2. Place your hands either a few inches from your body, palms up, or resting on the baby area.
3. Let your feet hang out to the sides 12–14 inches apart. (Figure 8.1)

Figure 8.1 The Sponge Position.

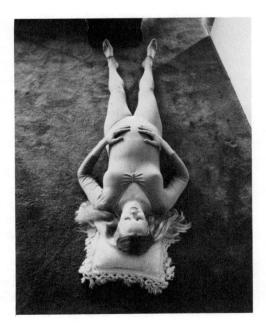

Cautions and Comments:

- This position should be discontinued after the seventh month. It may cause numbness to the legs because of the baby's weight cutting off the blood supply to the lower limbs.

- You may want to add another pillow under your knees for greater comfort.

- This position can also be practiced with your legs raised on an ottoman. (Figure 8.2)

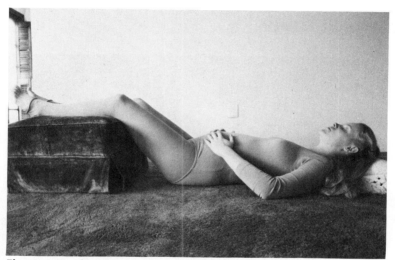

Figure 8.2 The Sponge with raised legs.

Side-Lying Relaxation Pose

Benefits:

- Increased comfort in the later and larger months of pregnancy
- Enables the body to completely relax
- Frees the spine from bearing any weight so that it can be relaxed
- Is an excellent sleeping position during the later months

Directions:

1. Lie on your left side, which is beneficial for your blood circulation. Place one pillow under your head and another one next to your legs on the inside. Bend your top knee and place it on the second pillow.

2. Place your hands in any comfortable position. Placing the top arm behind you is often helpful. (Figure 8.3)

Cautions and Comments:
- This is the most popular reclining position during the later months of pregnancy.
- You may want to add a third pillow near the middle of your back for extra comfort, or move the pillow near the legs up so that it fits under your abdomen. A pillow under the abdomen releases tension from the lower back.
- This is a popular breastfeeding position if you want to feed your baby while lying down.

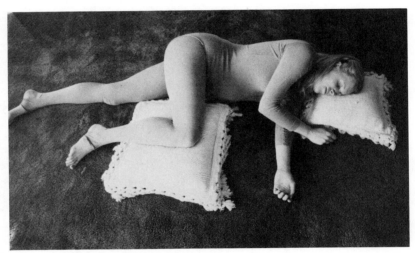

Figure 8.3 Side-Lying Relaxation pose.

Other Advisable Positions for Relaxation:

- Backward-Sitting Chair Position (See Chapter 13 for details)
- Sitting in a chair with your feet on an ottoman
- Cross-Legged Meditative Pose (see Chapter 9 for details)
- 45° Leg Rester (See Chapter 7, Part I for details)

The following posture, Complete Relaxation, may seem very simple to you as you read over the directions. You may think, "Oh, that's easy. This should be a snap to learn." Let me warn you before you begin that practicing this posture will take a lot of mental concentration. Your brain will try to divert you with more interesting tidbits and gossip. Don't get lost in your own idle thoughts while you try to practice this relaxation. If a thought comes in, let it pass; do not dwell on it as you then get back to the many steps involved in learning how to relax your body at will. With consistent mental and physical practice, you will master this all-important pose. Mastery of it will contribute to a more positive pregnancy, birth and motherhood experience.

Complete Relaxation

This can be practiced in a variety of relaxation poses. Breathe inhaling through the nose and exhaling through the mouth.

Benefits:
- Deeply relaxes the muscles and nervous system
- Releases stored tensions and anxieties, thereby restoring a peaceful feeling to the body and the mind
- 20 minutes of Complete Relaxation is equal to two hours of sleep
- Is a useful energizer
- Prepares the pregnant woman for the relaxation periods between con-tractions
- Helps to keep your blood pressure within normal range

Directions:
Variation I: Contract, Release, Relax

1. Settle into a comfortable relaxation position.
2. Take two to four "Rock-the-Baby" breaths to get centered.
3. Close your eyes. Contract all the facial muscles. Try to move all the facial muscles toward the nose and feel the tightness. Hold five seconds. Release. Breathe.
4. Squeeze the shoulders up around your neck and feel the tightness. Squeeze harder. Hold five seconds. Release. Breathe.
5. Make fists with the hands and tighten the arms. Tighten harder as you raise them a few inches. Hold five seconds. Release. Breathe.
6. Push the shoulder blades together. Squeeze harder. Hold five seconds. Release. Breathe.
7. Contract the buttocks and feel the tightness. Squeeze harder. Hold five seconds. Release. Breathe.
8. Tighten the thighs, knees and calves. Feel the tightness. Hold five seconds. Release. Breathe.

9. Push your heels away from the body by pointing the toes toward the knees as you feel the tightness. Hold five seconds. Release. Breathe.

10. Open your mouth wide as you inhale and sigh out the breath: a-a-a-h. Repeat five times.

11. Focus your concentration on your facial muscles and feel the forehead and eyebrow area going limp. Make that area let go even more.

12. Mentally focus on your eyes. Relax your eyes.

13. Feel your jaw muscles and cheek muscles let go. Feel the looseness. Separate your teeth and let your tongue fall back slightly into your mouth. Feel the muscles in the mouth area letting go.

14. Feel your nostrils, ears, and scalp relaxing.

15. Let all expression melt from your face. Feel it going limp.

16. Relax the neck: the front, the sides, the back of the neck.

17. Feel your shoulders letting go: the right shoulder, the left shoulder, and the space between.

18. Feel your upper arms, elbows, lower arms relaxing.

19. Feel your fingers opening slightly and releasing.

20. Feel your chest and back going limp. Feel the top half of your body completely relaxed and loose.

21. Relax the tummy area to give the baby more room. Feel the inner abdominal muscles letting go.

22. Feel your buttocks going limp, letting go.

23. Focus in on the birth canal area and feel it loose and relaxed. Check to see that your mouth is still relaxed. Relax the mouth and the birth canal.

24. Feel your thighs, hips, knees, calves and ankles going limp.

25. Feel your feet letting go. Make your toes relax one by one.

26. Take a moment or two to check your body over for further tension.

27. Feel yourself sinking into the mat or the chair. Let go, give up. Feel a sense of looseness enveloping you.

28. Feel the tensions draining out of your fingers and your toes. Imagine a flow of tensions, tiredness, troubles, fears, anxieties, and aches leaving your body as you open all the muscles.

29. Let your breathing settle down to a comfortable rate as you sink into the blissful feeling of complete relaxation.

30. Allow your consciousness and your baby's consciousness to connect. Let yourself be open to receive any feelings from your child.

31. Try to keep your mental awareness on your child as you relax for ten to 20 minutes.

32. When rousing out of a Complete Relaxation, take your time.

33. First get your awareness on how your body feels. Become aware of your hands and legs. Move your fingers slowly, then your toes, then begin to stretch and slowly rouse.

34. Walk yourself up into a sitting position using your hands if you are practicing lying down.

35. You should feel revitalized and reenergized after your practice.

Variation II: Release, Relax

1. Once you have mastered Variation I and find that you can relax your muscles at will, you can eliminate the muscle contraction part of this preceding posture.

2. You can begin your practice with #10.

Cautions and Comments:

- This posture is much easier if someone else with a soothing voice reads the directions to you. Your husband or a friend may be able to help you out or you can tape the directions for practicing.

- I have prepared a Complete Relaxation practice tape which is listed in the Appendix.

- Do not be discouraged if it takes you a full 20 minutes just to get all your muscles to relax. Keep practicing until your body responds to your mental commands.

- Try not to fall asleep during this relaxation. Rather go into a deep relaxation or a light meditative state with mental clarity.

- See Chapter 9 for a variety of topics on which to mentally focus when you practice Complete Relaxation.

Nine

Concentrations and Meditations for Inner Bonding

When women are pregnant, there is a natural tendency to pay more attention to what is going on inside their bodies. There are daily physical and mental changes to be recognized and necessary adjustments to be made. You may find yourself daydreaming about what your baby will be like; whether you will be a "good" mother; how labor will be, etc. This turning inward is a natural and, in most cases, enjoyable aspect of impending birth. Since your thoughts are dwelling with the baby, it is natural and quite beneficial for you to learn how to practice concentrative and meditative processes which can increase and deepen your pregnancy experience while developing your mental skills as well.

Within the last few years the medical community has begun to realize the vital part that bonding plays in the parent-child relationship. Bonding means that you and your mate share the first minutes and hours of your new baby's life. It means holding and playing with your baby immediately upon his or her arrival. The emotional tie that develops during this time has a very beneficial influence on the relationship that the parents share with the child in future years.

Since your baby's consciousness is developing and you are inwardly-oriented due to the pregnancy state, it is only logical that you can practice a pleasant form of "inner bonding" while you are awaiting your first encounter, or "outer bonding," with your baby. You may naturally be doing this anyway. To encourage this mental preparation for having a baby, some very enjoyable concentrations and meditations have been developed.

Using your imagination to create different scenes and experiences, often including your future child, is the basis of these mental exercises. These mental trips will strengthen the tie that you have with your child as well as teach you how to control your brain. It takes some mental effort to experience these concentrations, but the time you spend disciplining your brain will give you very tangible rewards: peace of mind, a positive attitude toward life, and, most of all, a warm anticipation of your new and future child.

Scientists have recently been studying what babies sense and how they feel inside the womb. The latest conclusion (which is not based on exhaustive study) is that babies are in a state of euphoria during the developmental time inside. All of their bodily needs are being taken care of by the mother's body, leaving the infant free to experience movement, sounds, feelings, intuition, and bliss. By using a Complete Relaxation and then a mental concentration, you can learn to share this bliss with your baby. Although your body is automatically doing the work of providing for your baby, your consciousness has to be trained to mentally link with your child.

The following mental concentrations should be used in partnership with a Complete Relaxation. It is only in a truly relaxed state that you can really delve into a concentration and thoroughly enjoy it. If you haven't practiced Complete Relaxation (pp. 155–57) take the time to do that before you try any of the following concentrations. You will find that it takes an inner determination to mentally complete a concentration. If your mind wanders while you are practicing, when you become aware of it, bring your attention back to the exercise. You may have to practice each exercise several times in order to do it from beginning to end. Having someone else read you the instructions may be quite helpful. If you make a Complete Relaxation tape for yourself, you can easily add any one of these concentrations to it.

CONCENTRATIONS FOR "INNER BONDING"

Sharing Your Baby's Present Home

1. Go through all the steps for a Complete Relaxation (pp. 155–57).

2. Focus your mental awareness on a beautiful beach near a calm warm lagoon of water. See all the details in the scene: the color of the sand, the trees, the sky, the water. Try to hear the sounds on your private island and realize that you are alone.

3. Imagine yourself walking into the water. Feel the water all over your body. Splash some water on your face.

4. Move around in the water. It is perfectly clear, safe, warm water with no dangerous fish or animals in it.

5. Feel the weightlessness of your body, your ease of movement in the water as your tiredness and tensions are washed away.

6. Realize that your baby is feeling the same way at this moment that you are in your imagination.

7. Open yourself to your child and let your feelings blend as you share your baby's home inside of you.

8. Remain in this pleasant state for several more minutes. If negative thoughts cross your mind, simply let them go and return to the feelings in the warm water.

9. When you wish to rouse, feel your body and then move your fingers and your toes. Finally begin to stretch.

10. Take one to two minutes to completely reawaken. You will feel refreshed and renewed and in closer contact with your child.

The Golden Ray of Sunshine

1. Do a Complete Relaxation until you are relaxed in a comfortable position.

2. Imagine that you are lying on a white beach on your own special island. This island is a magical place and all kinds of wonderful things can happen here.

3. Feel a special golden ray of sunshine shining down on you. This sunshine will not burn you in any way. It has healing, tension-releasing, and rejuvenating powers.

4. Feel the sunshine on your outer body. Feel it on your face, your chest, your arms, fingers, your legs, and your feet.

5. Feel the warmth all over the baby area of your body.

6. Now imagine this special sunshine going right through your skin and inside of you.

7. Feel this healing light inside of your head melting away your worries.

8. Feel this special light inside of your chest, inside of your arms, your hands, your legs, your feet, and your buttocks.

9. Feel this shiny golden light warming and preparing your birth canal area.

10. Now imagine this special light encircling your baby like a big golden bubble.

11. Let your baby be bathed in this golden bath of healing light.

12. Feel your whole being and that of your baby being energized with a golden light.

13. Remain in this golden light for several moments. Enjoy the feelings of inner warmth and protection when you are in this light.

14. Rouse slowly and deliberately when you want to get up. Take one to two deep breaths and slowly rouse your hands and feet, then the rest of your body.

Opening up to Bliss

This concentration is based on some personal correspondence I have had with Frederic Leboyer, the author of the beautiful book, *Birth Without Violence*. Mr. Leboyer is concerned with improving the baby's birth experience by encouraging a quiet atmosphere when the baby is born and then immersing the newborn in a warm water bath. This water bath duplicates the feeling and surroundings the baby had inside the womb and gives the child a secure and familiar feeling. Mr. Leboyer and I both believe in the importance and benefits of inner bonding. If you open yourself up to your child, you can receive the message that your child has to offer while it is living inside of you. This concentration can help you to do that.

1. In any comfortable position, practice Complete Relaxation until you are fully relaxed.
2. Center your awareness on the baby growing inside of you. See if you can feel the baby at this moment.
3. Now consciously quiet your mind by concentrating on your breath coming in and going out for several minutes. Let your breathing settle down.
4. Begin to dwell with your child as you imagine your whole being opening up to him or her.
5. Let the bliss, the contentment, the protection, the happiness, the love that your baby feels and lives with at this moment, pour into you.
6. Imagine a secret doorway through which these wonderful feelings can pass to you. Open the doorway a bit wider so that you can be flooded with these good and satisfying feelings.
7. Accept that your child can give to you, just as you give and will continue to give to your child.
8. Immerse yourself in these good feelings for a few more moments.
9. Then rouse slowly and conscientiously to retain any remnant of these pleasurable feelings.

The Baby's Birth Trip

This concentration is based on a discussion I once had with my two sons. I asked them if they could remember how it felt to be born. My older son, Mathew, who was seven years old at the time, did not have any strong recollections. However, my younger son, Michael, who was four years old, said he could remember. "It felt," he said, "like a lot of people were stepping on me at the same time." I was intrigued with his answer, and from it came the realization that the birth trip is a dual and rough process. During birth you are very aware that your body is physically moving your baby into this world. But your baby is encountering a different type of trip as it is squeezed and pushed to be born. The following concentration should give you a better understanding of what your baby will be going through during its birth. Hopefully it will encourage you to mentally talk to and reassure your child all during the labor process. That mental connection will benefit both of you.

1. Do a Complete Relaxation (pp. 155–57).

2. Take two to three "Rock-the-Baby" breaths to center yourself and bring your awareness to your child.

3. Concentrating on your baby, use your imagination to make believe that you are the baby for a few moments.

4. Imagine how your baby feels all warm, all wet, quite contented and blissful. Become the baby as you imagine that you feel your arms and legs tightly closed next to you. Feel the softness of the conforming walls all around you.

5. Imagine the regular thumping of the blood pulsing by. Hear the other noises surrounding this warm, compact home.

6. All of a sudden begin to feel the soft walls getting harder and squeezing you, then squeezing you even harder. Then they release and there is a return to the usual feelings.

7. Continue to feel the walls tightening around you squeezing you again, but for a longer period of time. "When will this end?" you are thinking. Then the squeezing stops only to begin again.

8. Now there is a new sensation: a feeling of great pressure from behind pushing, pushing, pushing even harder.

9. You are being pushed down a narrow, dark, warm tunnel. Feel yourself being pushed forcefully down, only to slide back up again. In your consciousness hear your mother reassuring you that she is with you and will protect you. Feel another push and great pressure behind you.

10. Sense that this black tunnel has an opening and you are getting near to it, as you feel great pressure on your face. Hear another message from your mother saying this trip is almost over.

11. Finally with a great force, your head is pushed through the end of the tunnel into a new place. It is bright, there are new noises. Feel some pressure on your head as someone touches it and guides you out.

12. Feel several more strong pushes as you are squeezed out of the tunnel. Feel warm hands holding you.

13. All of a sudden there is a warm, soft place below you and you can hear that familiar heartbeat once again. It reminds you of the place you used to be in.

14. Feel warm, protected and loved on your mother's tummy. Be thankful that the birth trip is over.

15. Now shift your concentrations away from that imaginary trip to your baby inside, who is going to make a very similar trip when the right time comes.

16. Reassure your child that you will be there with him or her all during the birth trip. You will be waiting expectantly to meet, love, hold and cuddle this new baby. Mentally discuss this and other feelings with your child for a few moments.

17. Rouse yourself when you find your mind is drifting.

18. Wiggle your fingers and feel them move. Just as your baby inside feels his or her fingers move. Feel your toes moving. Stretch and feel your feet just as your baby does.

19. Come back to this level of awareness with a better understanding of what is coming for your child and the very vital role you will play in this experience.

PREGNANCY MEDITATION

The preceding concentrations have exercised your powers of creation, imagination, and centering. At other times you may want to practice yoga meditation, which is a deeper form of concentration. The meditational practices within this book are quiet, repetitive practices to allow you to experience another state of consciousness: the meditation state. Within this state your perceptions and feelings may change. Often it is difficult to remember just what happened during your meditation, when you return to this level of consciousness. Meditation is a tool for learning to discipline the mind just as the asanas are a tool for learning to discipline the body. The bound elephant which appears on the Acknowledgement page pictorially represents the still and peaceful mind during meditation. Practicing meditation will give the body and brain the highest level of rest possible. Usually after a 20-minute meditation period you will feel energetic and peaceful.

Your spine must be straight in order to get into a meditational state; therefore you must sit up to meditate. You can sit in a comfortable cross-legged position (Figure 9.1) with a pillow under your buttocks for added comfort. Sit next to a wall if your back is not strong. You can sit on a

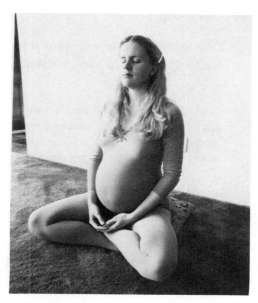

Figure 9.1 Cross-legged meditation position with a pillow.

Seiza Bench (p. 121) or in a comfortable chair with an ottoman and no head support. Your hands should be placed loosely in your lap or on the baby area. Do not clasp your hands. Placing the back of the right hand lightly on the palm of the left is a very useful hand position.

It is helpful to practice your prenatal asanas for ten to fifteen minutes before you practice meditation. This will limber your body, release tension and ensure that you will be able to sit still for a determined period of time. Mentally decide that you will be leaving your present situation to find an inner peace. Anticipate that you will find a peaceful feeling and will share it with your baby.

Always begin your meditation period with some form of controlled breathing. The following breaths would be the most advantageous: Alternate Nostril breath (pp. 16–18), 10 rounds; "Rock-the-Baby" breath (pp. 13–14), 10–15 breaths; or Smooth Breath (pp. 20–21), 10 breaths. Do not skip the breathing or you may have a difficult time relaxing.

Use the following meditation for a 20 minute period twice a day. Choose a quiet place where you will not be disturbed to meditate.

Baby Meditation
(Meditation with a Mantra)

This must be practiced in a sitting position.

Benefits:
- Allows the body to settle into a deep, relaxed state and eliminate deep tensions

- Enables the body to function more efficiently
- Practiced on a daily basis, heightens the senses

Directions:

1. Close your eyes, settle into a comfortable sitting position, and do the recommended rounds of breathing. Part by part do a complete bodily relaxation, and begin to focus your attention. You will be using the word "BABY" as your mantra.

2. Slowly start to inhale as you *mentally* think the syllable *ba* (bay) and then follow it with an exhalation as you think the syllable *by* (bee). Continue to think *ba* as you inhale and *by* as you exhale.

3. Allow your breathing to slow down as you continue to concentrate on those two sounds.

4. If your mind wanders, bring it back to sounds of *ba* when you inhale and *by* when you exhale. When other thoughts come in, as they will, brush them aside and go back to the sounds.

5. Continue to coordinate these mental sounds with your breathing for the duration of the meditation. Be sure to keep your head up straight and stay perfectly still.

6. When your 20 minutes is over (you can peek at your watch to see), bring your hands over your eyes and take two to three deep breaths.

7. Slowly stretch, rouse, and move.

8. See how refreshed and calm you feel.

Cautions and Comments:

- Using sounds as your seed for meditation is a form of Mantra Yoga. A mantra is a special sound which helps to calm and center the mind and body. If you have been practicing TM (Transcendental Meditation) and you have your own mantra, by all means continue to use it all during your pregnancy.

- The repetition of the mantra sounds has a calming and hypnotic effect on the brain and body.

- Your breathing will slow down and become more shallow as you get more into the meditation. Your body will still be receiving more than adequate amounts of oxygen because bodily efficiency increases during meditation.

- Do not let your head fall forward while meditating. Always keep your eyes closed.

- Try to sit for the entire 20 minutes. If you change positions go back to meditation as soon as you are settled.

- Always wait at least two hours after eating to meditate.
- Allow the peacefulness to fill you and the baby.

Mental Traps While Meditating:

1. I have an itch on my foot and I have to scratch it.
2. I think I may have left the stove on; I had better stop this meditation and go and look.
3. I am doing so well, I am having no thoughts at all. I am concentrating on my breath.
4. I think my body is going numb. What if I can't move when I try to . . .
5. I wonder if the latest story about so-and-so is really true? Is he saying those kinds of things now? Oh, no, that can't be true.

Listed above are some of the many mental diversions your brain will find for you while you are concentrating on your mantra. I am sure your brain will create others which will intrigue you even more. When these thoughts come into your brain, you must learn to brush them aside and simply go back to the point of concentration. If you have an itch, scratch it and immediately return to meditating. Sitting still and quiet is often frustrating in the beginning, but as you continue to practice, it will become easier. If you are thinking about how nice it is to meditate, you are not meditating!

The only way to learn how to meditate is to practice daily until you have trained yourself to do it. It is often helpful to join a yoga meditation class to help your progress. See if you can find one to your liking in your town.

The information contained in this chapter is meant to introduce you to the topic of concentration and meditation, so that you can include them in your daily practices. These mental disciplines complement the physical aspect of the yoga prenatal program. (For more information on meditation books, check the bibliography under "Meditation.") Once you practice and master these concentration and meditation states, you can put yourself into them at will. This ability is invaluable during labor and delivery as well as during other times in your daily life.

Ten

The Physiology
of Birth

Within the warm, dark, soft, wet inner reaches of your being at one unnoticed moment in time, a new consciousness begins its journey into life. Conception is truly one of nature's miracles. Each month within your body an ovum, or mature egg, 1/125th of an inch is released from your ovary. The egg must make a ten-day journey to the cavity of the uterus more than three inches away. The approach which the egg must take is through the Fallopian tube, where the lining is wrinkled unevenly and the passageway at the inner end is no larger than a bristle. The ovum must make this journey with no means of locomotion. It must depend on external methods for propulsion. A stream of fluid in the tubes, tiny hairlike projections, and the muscular motion of the Fallopian tubes themselves, propel the tiny ova toward the uterus. When the ovum is scarcely a third of the way down the tube, the grand event occurs: it meets a sperm and a new human being is begun! The genetic material of the father is added to that of the mother when fertilization takes place, usually in about an hour. Immediately after fertilization, early cell division results in a solid ball of cells which resembles a raspberry and is called "morula." This growth occurs during the 96 hours after conception. Cell division continues and the cell mass develops two distinct regions: an outer layer of cells which will form the placenta, and an inner ball of cells within which is the embryo and which will become a fully developed baby. The cell mass implants itself into the uterine wall after a seven-day journey down the Fallopian tube and into the uterus. This is the time in the monthly cycle when the lining of the uterus has reached its greatest thickness. The nesting cluster of cells continues to multiply and transform rapidly. As the months slip by the baby grows and develops. There are some other changes which are occurring within your body which may surprise you:

- Your total blood volume increases from 30–60 percent during pregnancy.
- As a result, the heart has to pump 50 percent more blood per minute when you are pregnant.
- The lungs are under pressure from the uterus, but your rib cage will widen to help compensate for this.
- The pregnant woman breathes much more air than the nonpregnant woman.
- The digestive system is not as efficient due to the growing uterus.

It should be obvious from these changes how beneficial controlled breathing and physical asanas can be during your pregnancy.

LABOR AND BIRTH

Labor is the climax of the maternity cycle. It is the process by which the fetus (baby) travels from the nest of the uterus to the outside world. The pictures below will depict this process which begins with "lightening" and is completed by expelling the afterbirth or placenta.

Lightening

Information and Tips:
- The baby descends lower into your pelvic area.
- You may find after the baby has dropped, it is easier to breathe, but you urinate more frequently.
- You may walk around in this condition for several days or weeks.

How Yoga Helps:
- Keep practicing the asanas, especially Salute to the Child, to keep your body in top shape for the impending birth.
- Increase your practice of Baby Breath to facilitate the pushing part of labor.
- Practice the Breathing for Birth Breaths.
- Do a 15–20 minute Complete Relaxation each day.

First Stage of Labor:

Information and Tips:
- The baby's head has moved more deeply into the pelvic outlet.
- The cervix has thinned and is beginning to dilate or open. It must

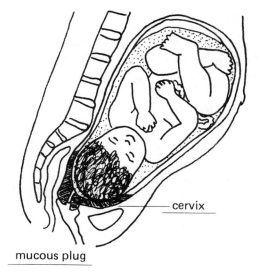

cervix

mucous plug

Figure 10.1 Lightening: Baby at zero station waiting for labor to begin.

Figure 10.2 First stage of labor: Cervix is opened 5 cms.

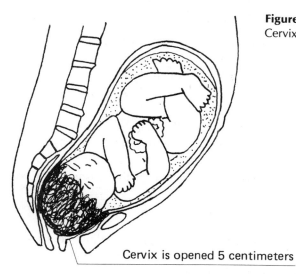

Cervix is opened 5 centimeters

open a full ten centimeters (four inches) for this part of labor to be over.

- The cervix must open wide enough for your baby's head to be pushed out.

How Yoga Helps:
- Use your Yogic Breathing for Birth techniques (pp. 185–86). Follow your coach's directions.
- Use an outside focal point for concentration.
- Completely relax all voluntary muscles between contractions.

171

- Keep in mental contact via an inner dialogue with your baby offering reassurance that you will be there to hold and to love the baby once the birth experience has ended.

Transition: the Late First Stage of Labor

Information and Tips:
- The cervix is nine centimeters dilated or opened and the baby's head is beginning to rotate.
- You may be having irrational thoughts and feelings at this time. You may feel ready to give up, get very hot or very cold and possibly shaky.
- The baby will be born very soon.

How Yoga Helps:
- Continue to use your Breathing for Birth techniques. (pp. 186–87)
- Pay strict attention to your coach as the breathing rhythm is switched.
- Keep your mental contact with the baby (between contractions), who is experiencing these strong contractions as well as you.
- Have coach massage lower back to eliminate pain.
- Use Blowing Breath if you have a premature urge to push.

Second Stage of Labor (Pushing):
- The opening of the cervix is completed and you can begin to push through each contraction.
- You may wonder where you get the energy for this pushing, but you will have it!

How Yoga Helps:
- All the squatting and pelvic loosening exercises will allow your pelvis to open its widest. Your child's head will fit so snugly that any bit of extra space will help you greatly at this time.
- If you have practiced your Pregnancy Sit-ups it will pay off now.
- Use Pushing Breath (pp. 193–94)
- Relax completely between pushes.

Crowning

Information and Tips:
- With your pushing through each contraction, the baby's head will finally be delivered.
- You may feel it as a burning and/or stretching sensation.

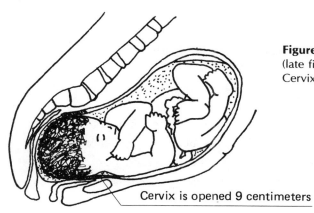

Figure 10.3 Transition (late first stage of labor): Cervix is opened 9 cms.

Cervix is opened 9 centimeters

Mother pushing

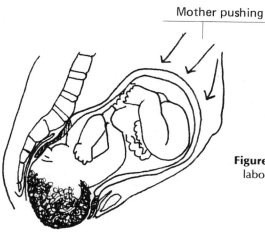

Figure 10.4 Pushing (second stage of labor): Mother pushing her baby out.

Figure 10.5 Crowning: The baby's head is being born.

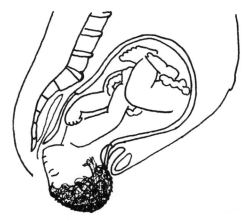

How Yoga Helps:
- You will need to use the Blowing Breath right after the baby has crowned to slow down the delivery of the rest of the child.

173

Rotation of the Head:

Information and Tips:
- After the birth of the baby's head, he or she will turn to one side or another with no aid.
- This allows the shoulders to be born one at a time.
- Once the shoulders are born, the infant's body will quickly follow.
- You will have to use the Blowing Breath to keep from pushing.
- Keep your mental dialogue with the baby going through the final phases of birth.

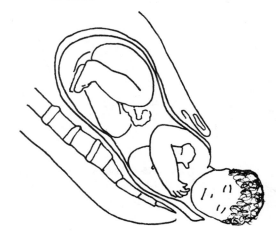

Figure 10.6 Rotation of the head: Baby turns as shoulder is born.

Third Stage of Labor (Expulsion of the Afterbirth):

Information and Tips:
- Pushing through several more contractions will expel the afterbirth.
- Afterbirth contractions also serve to reduce uterine hemorrhage.

How Yoga Helps:
- You will have to breathe and push through several more contractions.
- Make your mental dialogue a verbal one by welcoming your baby to this world!!

Although the drawings and descriptions within this chapter will help you visualize what is going on inside your body during labor and delivery, they will fade from your memory once you have totally experienced the birth of your child. If you are faithful in your practice of yoga asanas, and breathing and relaxing techniques, your body will work beautifully for you and your baby.

Eleven

Massage for Pregnancy, Birth, and Parenthood

Massage can help to relax the body, and increase circulation, sensation, and energy while promoting a general sense of well-being. Besides all those very rational reasons: it feels great! Touching is a very powerful means of nonverbal communication between people. You should approach massage as a precious gift shared by two people: the giver and the receiver. Massage can add new dimensions to the relationship you share with your mate. The type of massage which is described and illustrated within this chapter can be used all during the pregnancy, labor, and the postpartum period. Massage in labor will depend on your personal birth experience. Developing a good massage relationship will help to heighten your sensual self. By tuning into your sensual self, you can more clearly and vividly experience all the things that happen in your life each day. This heightened sensitivity can add joy to your daily life.

SOME SIMPLE RULES FOR MASSAGE

1. When you are using different strokes during a massage, glide from one stroke to another as smoothly as you can.
2. Try to mold your hands to your partner's body contours.
3. Vary the speed and pressure of your strokes, but do so smoothly.
4. The person who is receiving the massage should be passive and should not try to help during the massage. The "receiver" should have eyes closed, the better to relax and enjoy the sensations.
5. Centering and tuning into the sensations of being stroked should be the receiver's main concern.

6. If massage is done for too long a time, in an irregular pattern, and without lubrication, you can actually make your partner more tense!

SPECIAL RESTRICTIONS FOR PREGNANT WOMEN

1. Women with varicose veins should not have their legs massaged. They should, however, elevate their legs during a massage.
2. Women who are suffering from toxemia should not be massaged at all.
3. The pregnant abdomen should only be very lightly massaged. Never put pressure or lie on it.
4. Women in the later months should not lie flat on their abdomen.

PREPARING FOR THE MASSAGE

1. Choose a warm, quiet place.
2. Massage on a carpeted floor on which you can place a blanket with an old sheet on top, in case you spill some oil. During the later months of pregnancy, it is often advantageous for the woman to sit with her legs open facing the back of an armless chair with the husband sitting in a chair facing her back. The woman may want to put her head on a pillow on the top of the chair.
3. You can buy massage oil, or use vegetable oil (safflower or coconut) to which you add some scented oil which is available in most health food stores in many scents. If you prefer not to use oil, use a scented talc instead. The oil or talc is to enable your hands to apply pressure and at the same time move smoothly over the surface of the skin. Store the oil in a plastic container with a closeable top and heat the bottle under hot water before using. *Note:* Vegetable oil will ultimately stain any towels with which it is in contact, so use old towels and sheets for massage.
4. The person who is receiving the massage should be nude. Keep a sheet or light blanket handy in case of coolness during the massage.
5. Make sure that your nails are short so as not to hurt your partner.
6. Light a candle or two and put on some soft music if you like. Try to make the atmosphere as intimate and soothing as possible.

MASSAGING THE BACK & SHOULDERS

This can be used during labor to induce relaxation.

1. Have the person who is to receive the massage get into a comfortable position. (Naomi, who is pictured in Figure 11.1, was sitting in the Zen Sitting Position with her head resting on an ottoman. David, her husband, is seen kneeling behind her in order to massage her back.)

2. Begin the massage by taking two to three "Rock-the-Baby" breaths together to get centered.

3. Squeeze some of the warmed oil onto your hands and rub them together until they are warm. Never pour the oil directly on the person who is receiving the massage.

4. Place your palms on the lower back and slowly, with some pleasant pressure, move your hands up to the shoulders on either side of the spine, across the shoulders, then back down along the sides of the back to the starting point. Try to get the oil evenly covering the whole back area. (Figure 11.1)

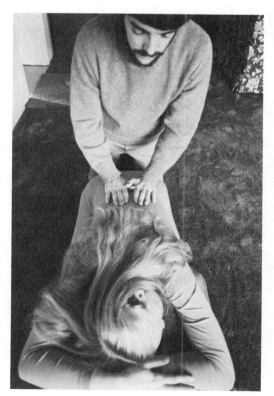

Figure 11.1 Main stroke to spread oil on back.

5. Use your fists to massage the lower part of the back (just above the crack in the buttocks). Use a circular motion on the buttocks and coccyx area. Check with your partner for a reaction. This area may need to be massaged during labor due to back labor. It is a good idea to practice massaging the spot well before labor, so that you are familiar with it. Your husband may find this movement tiring at first and will eventually begin to develop the muscles for a sustained massage for longer periods of time. (Figure 11.2) To relieve back labor, the coach can use fists or two tennis balls to apply lower back pressure. It is advisable during the last 6 weeks of the pregnancy for the coach to practice this part of the massage, since it can be quite tiring.

6. Once the lower back feels somewhat relaxed, move your attention to the waist area. This is an area of extreme tension and often pain during pregnancy. The person giving the massage should make a fist with the dominant hand, oil the lower arm, bend that arm at the elbow, then draw the entire lower part of the arm across the receiver's lower back. (Figure 11.3) Repeat the motion until the lower back is warm and relaxed.

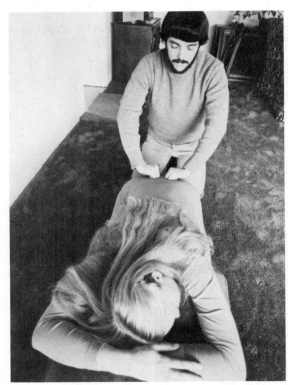

Figure 11.2 Fists massaging the lowest section of the spine.

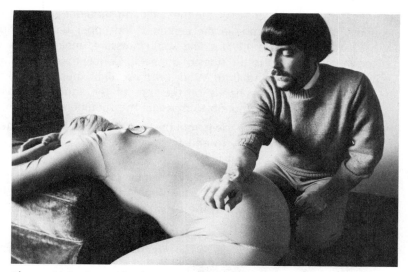

Figure 11.3 Lower back massage using the lower arm.

7. Placing the thumbs on either side of the spine (never, never massage directly on the spine), move the thumbs out with firm pressure to the sides of the body. (Figure 11.4) Work your way up the back with this motion or any other stroke that you and your partner like. You may want to use the same motion you used to spread the oil.

Figure 11.4 Thumbs massaging up the back next to the spine.

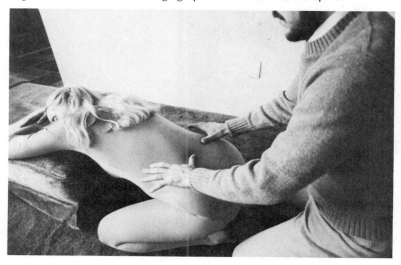

8. Once you are ready to massage the neck and shoulder area (a tension spot), place the thumbs in the center of the upper back and lower neck region. (Figure 11.5) Using some pressure, make circles with the thumbs moving to the sides of the neck. Concentrate on any areas which seem hard and firm. Work on these tight muscles until they loosen up. Move the hands on the tops of the shoulders, using a kneading or pinching motion to massage the shoulders.

9. Inventing some of your own motions for you and your partner to share is a wonderful way to enhance a massage.

10. To finish this massage, lightly place your fingertips on top of your partner's head and slowly and very lightly move your fingers down the back and to the buttocks area. Repeat this light effleurage three to four times as a signal that the back massage is over.

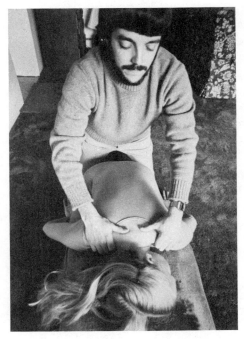

Figure 11.5 Massaging the neck and shoulder areas.

Parts of this basic massage may be used during labor for reducing muscle tension and inducing a more relaxed state. Many women do not like to be touched when they are laboring. Since each laboring experience is different, you will have to wait and see if you want to use this back massage. However, practicing can be a lot of fun!

Using mutual massage as a way of sharing pleasurable sensations and feelings can be most helpful, especially when making love is difficult or prohibited for a variety of reasons. Learning about how a person feels, how his muscles feel, how his bones feel, where he carries tensions, where he is loose and relaxed, etc., can deepen a mutual relationship. It is one of the most pleasurable ways to relax.

SELF-MASSAGE FOR ELIMINATING HEADACHES

This massage can be given to you by your mate as well.

When you feel a headache coming on, the first thing to practice is Alternate Nostril Breathing which will often eliminate the headache before it really gets painful. However, if you have a full-blown headache, the following head, neck, and shoulder massage should prove quite useful.

1. Wash your hands. Begin the massage by taking two to three "Rock-the-Baby" breaths. Place your fingers on your forehead above your eyebrows and massage across that area with moderate pressure until you come to the temples. Massage the temples and behind the ears, then down the neck to the shoulders. (Figure 11.6) Repeat three times increasing your pressure as you go.

2. Place your dominant pointer or third finger on the top of your head and look for sensitive points. Often they will be across the top of your head going from the front of your head to the back. (Figure 11.7) Work these sensitive spots with firm pressure until the knot dissolves or the pain subsides. Work all the painful places.

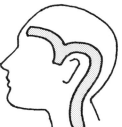

Figure 11.6   Areas to be massaged to eliminate headaches.

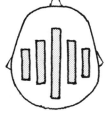

Figure 11.7   Sensitive areas to be worked on the top of the head.

3. Next check the back of your neck where it connects to your head. Find any sensitive areas in this region (Figure 11.8) and work them with your thumbs, index or middle fingers until the pain subsides.

Figure 11.8 Sensitive areas at the back of the neck.

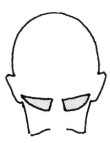

4. Do two to three Neck Rolls to release tension.

5. Check the neck now and massage any tight areas. Find the sensitive areas and massage until the pain subsides.

6. Check the shoulders now. You may want to shrug them several times. Place your right hand on your left shoulder and firmly squeeze along the top of the shoulder until it joins the arm. Do the same thing on the other side. If the shoulders are still not loose, repeat two to three more times.

7. Finish with ten rounds of Alternate Nostril Breath.

Twelve

Breathing
for Birth

Natural and rhythmic breathing with an inner or outer focal point is necessary for a happier and less tiring labor and delivery. You already know that learning to work with the flow of the body is an essential part of practicing asanas. This training is invaluable in labor because working with the natural rhythms of your laboring body will help to speed the process to its natural conclusion: the birth of your child. If you have been practicing yogic breathing during your pregnancy, you already have experienced the calming and rejuvenating effects it can have on you. During labor, controlled and rhythmic breathing serves two purposes. First, it keeps the body filled with needed energy for its hard work. Second, it becomes one focal point on which you pin your awareness.

If you have been practicing yogic breathing techniques, you should have very few problems adapting to breathing for birth. Yogic Breathing for Birth is very similar to the techniques which are taught in the Lamaze natural childbirth classes. If you are able to take a series of prepared childbirth classes with your husband or a friend, you will find that this kind of training will be exceedingly helpful during your labor. Having a coach to monitor your breathing during labor will help you to keep in control. However, some of my students are, for a variety of reasons, not able to take any other classes than prenatal yoga. They have been able to utilize the following techniques throughout their labors. One student who had her first baby without any drugs, in two hours and 25 minutes said that yogic breathing really worked!

In order for these breathing techniques to work for you, you *must* practice them daily with your coach for ten to fifteen minutes during the last six weeks of your pregnancy. If you are not able to take any prepared childbirth classes, explain these techniques to your coach who can be your husband or a friend. Have your coach check to see that you are relaxed and rhythmic in your breathing while you practice and during labor. The more familiar you become with these breaths, the more useful and natural they will be for you during your hours of labor.

An inner or outer focal point is highly beneficial for easing you through each contraction. Some outer focal points which are helpful include

- the eyes of your coach, which can be very powerful
- a spot on the wall or ceiling, which can get rather dull
- a picture you really like to look at
- a religious symbol, if it makes you feel protected and helped
- a Birth Mandala, (Figure 12.1) which should keep your interest

During each breathing series, you should keep your concentration on your outer focal point as you breathe.

An inner focal point may be of help for any time during the labor you feel yourself going inward. Mentally chanting "Om," the universal sound, is

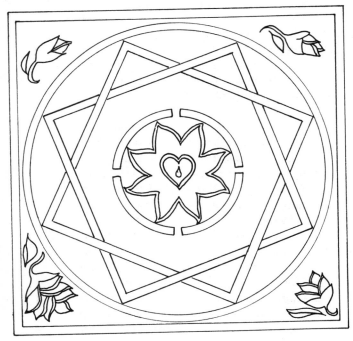

Figure 12.1 This special birth mandala can be used for outward concentration during your laboring time. Make a copy of it, color it, and pack it in your bag to take to the hospital (or use it at home).

extremely powerful (it is mentally chanted: O-O-O-M-M). However, you must not focus on the contraction or you may lose control. Practicing your Breathing for Birth exercises with your coach will help you prepare for the hours during labor that you will share. The latest medical research indicates that women who go through labor with their husband or a friend coaching have a more positive experience and often a shorter labor.

Stages of Labor

It is wise to approach labor with the understanding that it has 3 basic parts. One section may go very quickly and uneventfully, while another section may prove full of complications. By mentally dividing it into sections, it will tend to seem shorter.

The most obvious symptom of early labor is a consistent pattern of contractions. The contractions may be uneven at first, but eventually they fall into a pattern. Contractions are usually 10–15 minutes apart at this time. Other symptoms of early labor are slight menstrual cramps, a bloody show or vaginal discharge (which is actually mucous tinged with pink rather than red), and possibly an inner feeling that the event you have been waiting for is actually beginning to happen. Many women experience the "nesting" instinct during the few days prior to the birth. You may find yourself washing floors, walls, cleaning out closets, and organizing your things in a sudden burst of energy. I remember quite well washing my kitchen floor 3 times during the three days prior to my first son's birth. It has never been that clean again!

Another very definite sign that labor is beginning is the breaking of your water bag which is experienced as a warm gush of water. You may think you are urinating, but you will find there is no way to control it. Placing a rolled hand towel between your legs is a good solution. You should call your doctor or midwife when these symptoms occur so that you can report on your progress. The following should be helpful to you for clarifying your understanding of labor.

STAGE ONE, EARLY LABOR

Characteristics:

1. Short, slight contractions
2. Ten to 15 minutes apart
3. May not cause discomfort
4. Your cervix is dilating or opening one to four centimeters. It has to open ten centimeters (4 inches) to go to Stage Two.

What to Do:

1. Keep moving about normally.
2. Practice Salute to the Child to center & stay limber.
3. Let your body tell you when to slow down or lie down.
4. Use "Rock-the-Baby" breath, (pp. 13–14) "Welcome-Farewell Breath," (pp. 188–89) and "Early Labor Breath." (p. 89)

STAGE ONE, ACTIVE LABOR

Characteristics:

1. Contractions three to five minutes apart, a more definite pattern
2. Your cervix is opening from four to eight centimeters (1½ to 2¼ inches)

What to Do:

1. Assume a comfortable position; try a variety of positions (see Chapter 13).
2. Change position frequently.
3. Listen to directions from your coach on breathing and relaxing.
4. Urinate every hour.
5. Use "Welcome-Farewell Breath" (pp. 188–89) and "Combined Breath" (p. 190) or any breathing pattern which is effective.
6. Do a "Complete Relaxation" (pp. 155–57) between contractions.
7. Mentally talk to the baby to report on the progress the two of you are making.
8. Keep your mouth relaxed throughout. Remember: "As the mouth goes, so goes the bottom."

STAGE ONE, TRANSITION

Characteristics:

1. Erratic and hard contractions
2. Two minutes apart or less
3. You may feel agitated, overwhelmed, or discouraged. These are wonderful signs, for it is almost time to push the baby out!

4. You may cry, feel a sense of panic, experience nausea, vomiting, sweating, coldness, rectal pressure, or the shakes.

5. Your cervix is opening from eight to ten centimeters or three to four inches.

6. This is the hardest but SHORTEST part of labor.

What to Do:

1. Use "Who-Ha Breath" (pp. 190–92) and "Blowing Breath." (p. 192)

2. Listen to your coach. Concentrate on outer or inner focus to keep control.

3. *Do not push* even if you have the urge: pant or blow instead.

4. Mentally keep telling yourself (and the baby, too) that this difficult stage will be over very shortly.

5. Try to be in the "here and now" by handling one contraction at a time. Do not anticipate the next one.

STAGE TWO, YOUR BABY'S BIRTH

Characteristics:

1. Strong contractions, but further apart and much less intense than during transition.

2. You may feel a very strong urge to push as you do when you have to move your bowels.

3. You may feel a burning sensation on the pelvic floor or a feeling of a giant bowel movement.

4. The uterine contractions combined with your pushing efforts will help your child to be born

What to Do:

1. Push when told, using "Pushing Breath." (pp. 193–94)

2. Relax your mouth and pelvic floor muscles.

3. Relax completely between pushes.

4. Pant or blow if you are told *not* to push.

5. Use an upright sitting or squatting position with support for best result.

6. Watch your baby being born!

STAGE THREE,
BIRTH OF THE PLACENTA

Characteristics:

1. Uterine contractions will continue after the baby is born.

2. If you have had an episiotomy, your doctor or midwife will be suturing it at this time. You will receive local anesthesia for this procedure.

3. Contractions may continue for a while and then slowly come to a stop.

What to Do:

1. Using "Pushing Breath," (pp. 193–94) push the placenta out.

2. Use any breathing technique you choose during subsiding contractions.

The state of consciousness right after the baby is born has been described by many women as "a super wonderful high." The body and the mind generate vast amounts of energy for your baby to arrive. Enjoy this heightened consciousness and excitement if it comes. If you have received drugs during your labor and delivery, you will most probably feel this "baby high" as well.

You will have to wait and see if any drugs will be necessary for your birth experience. Place your trust and faith in your doctor or midwife to guide you in this area.

If you approach labor as a positive experience for which you are well prepared and energized, you will be able to face all the challenges that come along. Labor means hard, long, sweaty, intense work. You are going to be hot; you are going to be tired; you may wonder if you will run out of energy. Do not go into labor with any preconceived notions such as "I will not take any medication," or "I know this labor is going to last forever," or "I know this is going to be easy as can be." Accept your laboring experience, work with it by using your breathing and having faith in your own inner strength.

BREATHS FOR LABOR AND BIRTH

Welcome-Farewell Breath

This can be practiced in any position.

Benefits:
- Mentally signals the beginning and the end of each contraction
- Keeps the body relaxed and well supplied with oxygen

Directions:

1. Keeping the facial and tummy muscles relaxed, inhale through the nose, rocking the baby forward.

2. Exhale slowly either through your nose or through a loosely opened mouth. Repeat.

Cautions and Comments:

- Treat each contraction as a unique experience or wave. Welcome it with a breath, breathe through it, and then say goodbye to it with a breath. Repeat.

- Keep these breaths slow, rhythmic, and even.

Early Labor Breath

This can be practiced in any position.

Benefits:

- Keeps the uterus and your body well supplied with oxygen

- Focuses your attention away from the contraction, thereby lessening your perception of pain

Directions:

1. As the contraction begins, take one or two Welcome-Farewell Breaths. Slowly inhale through your nose, sending the air to your chest area. Your tummy will move out, but keep your awareness on the chest area expanding forward with each inhalation.

2. As you inhale, think: "In, two, three, four, five." As you exhale, think: "Out, two, three, four, five."

3. Keep your breathing even and your focus on counting each breath, as well as on your outside focal point.

4. You should take six to ten Early Labor Breaths during each 60–second contraction.

5. Keep your mind at all times on your breathing and counting.

6. When the contraction is ending, do one or two Welcome-Farewell Breaths and resume normal breathing until the next contraction begins.

Cautions and Comments:

- Develop a comfortable inhalation and exhalation count.

- Keep your inhalations and exhalations smooth, even, and rhythmic.

- Try to use your nose for inhaling and exhaling.

Combined Breath (for mid-labor)

Benefits:
- Increases the need for concentration by changing the rate of the breath, thereby lessening the perception of pain
- Keeps the diaphragm up and away from the uterus during the peak of the contraction
- Keeps the body and the baby well supplied with energy

Directions:
1. When the contraction begins, take one or two Welcome-Farewell breaths. Use Early Labor breath until the contraction begins to peak and you need to switch to Mouth-Centered Breathing.
2. Mouth-Centered Breathing is shalllow in-out mouth breathing with an increased rate. The air is inhaled into the back of the throat and the upper part of the chest with a "who" sound and exhaled quickly but rhythmically with a "ha" sound.
3. When the contraction has peaked and begun to subside, return to Early Labor breath and finish the contraction with one or two Welcome-Farewell Breaths.

Cautions and Comments:
- This pattern will work well during the middle stages of labor when the cervix is opening from approximately three to seven centimeters (1½ inches to 2¾ inches).
- You must keep your mouth open and relaxed during Mouth-Centered Breathing
- You may want to invent your own patterns for using the Early Labor breath. You may want to inhale/exhale for 5, then reduce it the next time to 4, then 3, and so on.
- When using the "Who" or "Ha" sounds for Mouth-Centered Breathing, whisper the sounds. Concentrate instead on the rhythm of the "Who" & "Ha."
- The faster Mouth-Centered Breathing is not very comfortable when you first try it. With practice, you will learn to bring in just enough air to keep the body energized without feeling out of breath.

Who-Ha Breath

This breath is to be used during transition. It may be practiced in any position.

Benefits:
- Increased mental concentration for switching patterns keeps your awareness away from the forceful contractions.

190

- Keeps the diaphragm up and away from the contracting uterus, thereby facilitating your labor.
- Keeps your mind occupied at a time when you may want to give up and go home.

Directions:

1. Begin your contraction with one or two Welcome-Farewell breaths.
2. As the contraction heightens (which will be very quickly), begin to quietly say "Who-Who-Who-Ha" in a very rhythmic way as you do Mouth-Centered Breathing. The beats should be even with no stopping between each series.
3. Use the Who-Ha breath through the entire contraction and finish with one or two Welcome-Farewell breaths.

Variations:

To make the concentration more complicated, vary this breath by using the following patterns:

Who-Who-Who-Ha
Who-Who-Ha
Who-Ha
Who

or

Ha
Who-Ha
Who-Who-Ha
Who-Who-Who-Ha

or

4 Who's + 1 Ha
6 Who's + 1 Ha
2 Who's + 1 Ha, etc.
Reverse

or invent your own patterns.

Cautions and Comments:

- Contractions during transition will last anywhere from 60–90 seconds with very little time between. They seem to tumble on each other.

- This breathing will make your mouth exceedingly dry, and it is advisable to take ice chips between contractions.
- Your husband or friend can indicate via finger movements which beat you should be on. Total concentration on this breath is necessary in order to keep control.
- The transition period of labor completes the opening of the cervix and is the most intense section of labor for most women. At this point you may feel irritable and as if you want to throw in the towel and go home. You may feel nauseated, very cold or very hot, very emotional or very tired. You may not want your husband near you or touching you. You may find that you are in another state of consciousness during transition. You are—so experience it, for your baby will soon be born.

Blowing Breath

This breath is to be used during transition when you want to push but you have been told not to. It may be practiced in any position.

Benefits:
- Redirects and diminishes the pushing urge until the proper time
- Lets a variety of tensions and emotions out

Directions:
1. During a contraction while you are using the Who-Ha breath, you may want to bear down and push. This is inadvisable until the cervix is fully dilated. Instead, you can blow forcefully out of your mouth, as if you are blowing out several candles on a cake.
2. The breathing pattern would look like this: Welcome-Farewell → Who-Ha (repeated) → Blowing Breath → Who-Ha (repeated) → Welcome-Farewell.
3. Blow in short bursts and repeat all during the urge to push.

Cautions and Comments:
- Pushing during transition may tear your cervix and make the labor last longer.
- Blowing should be used only when you have the urge to push and may not. Panting may be substituted for blowing if you are more comfortable with it. You can pant by keeping the mouth slightly open and inhaling and exhaling quickly.

Pushing Breath

This should be done in squatting or partial sitting position for best results.

Benefits:
- Enables the body to bear down and push the baby through the birth canal and into this life
- Enables you to adequately utilize the oxygen which your system has at the moment

Directions:
1. As the contraction begins, in a relaxation position, take one to two Welcome-Farewell breaths. Exhale completely but quickly and then fill up with as much air as you can and hold your breath with your chin tucked into your chest.
2. You should be in a half-sitting or squatting position for this section of the breath. With your lungs full of air, open the birth canal (as in Baby Breath), bear *down* and push for a count of ten (Your coach should do the counting). Quickly exhale and inhale deeply again and repeat bearing down and pushing.
3. As the contraction begins to subside, return to a relaxation position; finish off with one to two Welcome-Farewell breaths.
4. Relax and breathe normally until the next contraction begins.

Cautions and Comments:
- You need to push down, up, and out, for that is the route your baby will take. Use your full lungs & abdominal muscles to push down.
- You have to think "down" as you push. Do not push in your face or you will burst blood vessels.
- You do not have to push with every contraction.
- You may be quite noisy when you push. This is fine.
- Push through your birth canal, not your anus. Pushing in the anal area causes postpartum hemorrhoids.
- You may hear the doctor, midwife, or nurses telling you to blow during the pushing stage, for they do not want your baby born too quickly. Use Blowing Breath during these sections of the pushing phase.
- You push with the same vaginal muscles you used in "Baby Breath." (pp. 14–16)
- You have to push during contractions to deliver the placenta out as well.

- Women having a second or third child will have afterbirth uterine contractions through which they will have to breathe for comfort.
- The baby will move down with each push and then slip back. At times it may seem frustrating. Finally the baby's head will leave the birth canal. Birth of the entire baby will follow very soon.

Thirteen

Advantageous Positions for Labor and Birth

You are not sick when you are in labor! You do not have to retire to your bed but are free to walk around, and move in and out of several positions during some of the time. Your freedom of movement is based to a great extent on where you choose to give birth. If you are having a home birth, you will obviously be able to move about as you and the circumstances permit. If you have a hospital birth, you may find that you have to stay in bed for the last part of the labor, especially if you have a birth monitor on your abdomen recording information about your baby. In either case, it is wise to become familiar with as many of the following laboring and birthing positions as you can. Many women have found that shifting out of an ineffectual position into a new position often speeds the progress of the labor and birth.

Laboring positions which tilt the torso forward utilize the force of gravity to help the laboring, pushing and birth process along. If you are in a conventional hospital setting, you may not be able to utilize some of the suggested pushing positions. If that is the case, follow the directions which you received in your prenatal education classes or from the hospital staff. If you are having a home birth with a midwife, you should become totally familiar with the pushing positions which are included here by practicing them during the last six weeks of your pregnancy. Shifting into a variety of positions makes labor *seem* shorter. Try practicing your Breathing for Birth breaths in all of these laboring positions so you can learn which positions are most comfortable. Many of the squatting and kneeling positions help to keep the pelvic and birth canal areas of your body in good tone.

HELPFUL POSITIONS
FOR THE EARLY AND MID
FIRST STAGE OF LABOR

1. Walking around and stopping for contractions
2. Lying down for resting or sleeping; use side lying position
3. Sitting and leaning on the back of a chair (Figure 13.1). Put a pillow on the top of the chair for comfort
4. Sitting in the Zen Sitting position with the knees open while resting on a chair (Figure 13.2)
5. Standing and leaning on the wall during contractions. Cradle your arms against the wall and rest your head on them
6. Squatting on heels or toes while holding onto a chair for support
7. Cross-legged sitting position (pp. 122–23)
8. Any other positions which you find comfortable

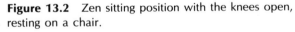

Figure 13.1   Sitting and leaning on the back of the chair.

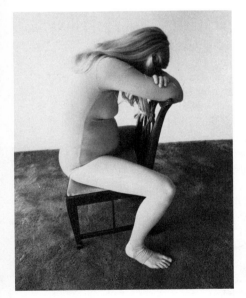

Figure 13.2   Zen sitting position with the knees open, resting on a chair.

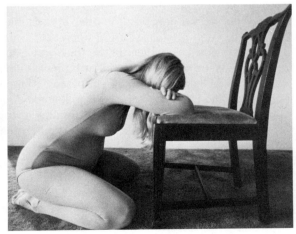

ADVANTAGEOUS POSITIONS
FOR LATE FIRST STAGE
OF LABOR (TRANSITION)

1. Kneeling onto a chair with the knees separated and the head up (Figure 13.3)

2. One leg bent and flat; other leg in a kneeling position. Arms rest on chair. Shift legs between contractions (Figure 13.4)

3. The Cat position with the back rounded a bit (#7 in Salute to the Child). Place your arms on a chair in this position if they get tired

4. Sitting and leaning forward

5. A semi-sitting, semi-reclining position with several pillows under your back. Your knees can be bent or you can have the legs flat. (This is the best position in bed)

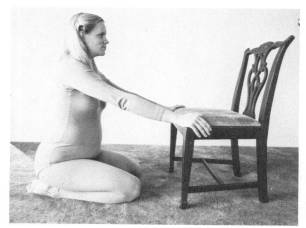

Figure 13.3 Kneeling (legs separated) next to a chair, with head up.

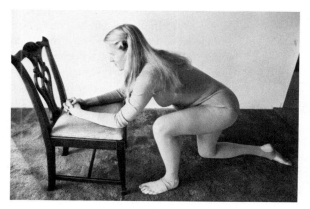

Figure 13.4 One leg kneeling, the other flat, and hands on chair.

USEFUL POSITIONS FOR THE
SECOND STAGE OF LABOR (PUSHING)

1. Squatting on toes or flat feet while bearing down holding onto a chair (Figure 13.5). You can lean your back against the wall in this position as well

2. Kneeling and leaning forward onto a chair for pushing (Figure 13.2)

3. The Cat Position (#7 in Salute to the Child)

4. Pushing in a semi-sitting reclining position with the legs open and knees bent. Have a wedge or some pillows behind you to retain this position. Place hands underneath knees, or place bent legs on bars on each side of the bed, or up in stirrups during the contraction to facilitate pushing

5. One leg kneeling, other leg flat, arms resting on a chair (Figure 13.3)

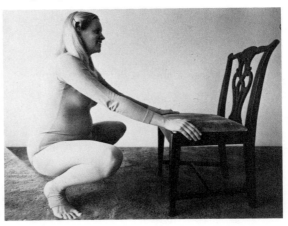

Figure 13.5 Squatting on toes near a chair.

These positions are only suggestions to which you can add your own. You will find that you will be changing position often during labor, so being familiar with a variety of movements can be helpful, especially during long labors. If you are in bed during labor, you can still go into some of the kneeling positions by turning sideways and using the bars on the sides of the bed for support. Do not use a flat back reclining position for labor and birth because it cuts your circulation and forces your body to work against gravity.

Introduce these different positions to your mate or coach before you go into labor. You may forget about many of these movements, but hopefully your coach will remember. Changing positions often will give you something else to think about during labor and delivery. A variety of laboring and birthing positions, controlled breathing and inner faith will help you to have a more positive birth experience.

Fourteen
A Primer for the Nursing Mother

Breastfeeding is the natural continuation of the physical union and compatibility which you have been experiencing during your pregnancy. It is merely a continuation of an involuntary process in a voluntary way.

The decision to breastfeed or bottlefeed your baby is a very personal one and should be shared with your mate. It is one of the first decisions you will make in your new parent roles. Many fine books have been written on this topic. (See the section on breastfeeding in the bibliography.) By doing some reading, and by talking to other women who have successfully nursed their babies, you will gather much information on which to base your decision. It is advisable to attend a local meeting of the La Leche League, which is a nonprofit organization concerned with teaching women how to successfully breastfeed their babies. Your doctor or midwife will probably have the name of your local group leader.

Medical research in this area has indicated that nursing your baby can be highly beneficial for the baby's growth and development, as well as for your own body. Some of the most important benefits of nursing are:

1. *Nutrition:* Your breast milk is perfect for fulfilling your baby's needs. It is raw and freshly made and can be rapidly and easily digested by your baby.

2. *Health:* Immunities to certain diseases for the first two years of the baby's life are contained in colostrum, which is produced during pregnancy and is consumed by the baby during the first few days until your milk comes in.

3. *Availability:* Breast milk is available immediately, at the right temperature, and in the right quantity wherever you and the baby are.

4. *Digestion:* The stools of breastfed babies are loose, mustard colored and have a mild odor. Rarely is there a problem with constipation.

5. *Economy:* Breast milk is economical and a great natural resource. You only have to add 1 additional serving of calcium foods and 500 calories daily to your well-balanced diet to produce more than enough milk for your baby.

6. *Relaxation:* The time that you and baby spend together during each feeding forces you to sit down, put your feet up, breathe deeply, and relax for good milk letdown and flow. This shared experience several times a day fosters a close physical and emotional relationship which can be enjoyed by both the mother and the baby.

If you have been persuaded to strongly consider nursing your baby, you should begin actively preparing both mentally and physically. Mental attitude regarding your breasts and the way you will be using them as a nursing mother has a very important bearing on your breastfeeding experience. The duality of the female body is most evident during pregnancy, birth, and lactation; during these times the primarily sexual parts of the body will be used for very different processes.

By accepting the very beautiful and utilitarian duality of your body, you may better adjust to the use of the breasts for nourishment of your child as well as for the sexual stimulation of your body during lovemaking. Since you really cannot entirely separate these two physical functions, you may feel somewhat sexually stimulated during the time you are doing nipple preparation. Accept these pleasurable feelings and enjoy them. You may feel sexual sensations while you are nursing your baby; these are a perfectly normal and natural part of a very close physical union or bond.

PRENATAL NIPPLE PREPARATION

Nipple preparation, especially for fair-haired women, can help to minimize sore nipples once the baby begins to nurse. It requires a few minutes of your time each day during the last three months of pregnancy. Learn to *gently* strengthen your nipples by doing the following:

1. Pull on your nipples by placing your thumb on the upper areola (brown part of the nipple) and your other fingers on the bottom of the aerola—pull out toward the nipple as the baby will when nursing. Repeat five to ten times.

2. Roughen your nipples with a towel after bathing or with a wet loofa sponge while showering. Rub vigorously but do not get into pain.

3. Do not use soap on your nipples. This will cause them to dry and crack.

4. Wear a supportive nursing bra during the last weeks of pregnancy. Air the nipples by opening the flaps.

5. Apply sesame oil or pure lanolin daily to soften the nipple area.

6. Put a piece of colored paper in your bathroom to remind you that every time you have to go to the bathroom, you should take a few moments for nipple preparation.

EQUIPMENT FOR BREASTFEEDING

One piece of equipment which will enhance your nursing experience is a rocking chair. The baby has been rocked all during its stay inside your body and the movement of a rocking chair can be very relaxing to both of you. The rocking chair that you choose should be high enough in the back to support your head and should have arms at the proper height to maximize comfort when you hold the baby. (Figure 14.1) Take your time when you are choosing a chair. Sit in each one for a few minutes until you find one which fits your body size and shape. A footstool or hassock is helpful so that you can put your feet up as you nurse. This benefits your blood circulation while adding to your comfort and relaxation.

Figure 14.1 Using a rocking chair while nursing the baby.

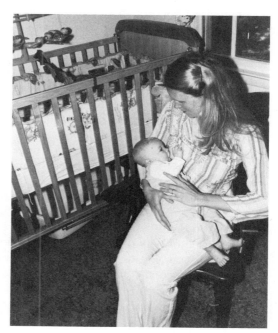

A second necessity for breastfeeding is a breast pump, which you can use to empty your breasts when they are too full or to pump out milk for future use. There are new pumps on the market which come with detachable bottles for easy and quick milk collection. One kind which is highly recommended is the Breast Milking and Feeding Unit available from the Happy Family Baby Products Company, 12300 Venice Blvd., Los Angeles, Calif. 90066; Telephone Toll Free #1–800–228–2021 Ext. 34. It is more expensive than most, but it works very well. Extra breast milk which you pump may be frozen (for up to two weeks) and then used at a later date.

MISCONCEPTIONS ABOUT NURSING

Many women believe they will be continuously tied to the baby if they breast-feed. However, many breastfed babies will take a bottle of previously pumped breast milk or formula when their mother is not available. There are many working women who just nurse their babies in the morning and evening and the baby is given formula during the day. The frequency of nursing is something that you and your baby can work out.

If you are out for the evening and your breasts become full, you can easily hand-express the extra milk in the nearest bathroom sink. If you have difficulty hand-expressing, you can carry your breast pump with you to eliminate the extra milk.

Another misconception is that you will not be able to make nutritious milk in adequate supply for your baby. You will be able to make enough nutritionally-balanced milk for your baby to grow and develop as long as you include 500 extra calories a day plus one extra serving of calcium rich foods in your postpartum diet, chosen wisely from the four main food groups. Your body will do the rest. Your natural "milk machine" will continue to supply your baby for as long as you and the baby choose.

Often small-breasted women question their ability to produce adequate supplies of milk. The size of the breast has very little to do with its ability to produce enough milk. Much of a woman's milk supply is stored in the back of her breasts. As the baby sucks out the front milk, the stored milk is drawn forward and consumed.

Before the invention of formula, women had little choice about breastfeeding their babies. It was an accepted part of the motherhood role. Learning about nursing and experiencing it even for a short time will deepen your understanding of how the female body functions. If you find that nursing is not right for you, you can easily put your baby on formula. Since you have both options open, the yogic approach would be the natural way first.

Fifteen

Three Personal Birth Stories

Reading someone else's birth story can be most helpful for preparing you for your own birth experience. Often a word or comment can give you more insight into the possibilities of the experience than reading books written about childbirth. The following three stories reflect a variety of options which are available to you at the present time.

HOME BIRTH

Pat and James McMullan chose to have their first child, Jason, at home. He was born on August 10, 1978, with three lay midwives attending. Pat tells their story:

The last two nights before Jason was born, I awoke several times with a feeling of heaviness deep in my abdomen. I would empty my bladder, but that would not really relieve the feeling.

I had felt well throughout my pregnancy and was not longing for it to end. Early in the morning on the ninth of August I felt "yucky" cramps that were like the worst period I had ever had—and for the first time I wanted the pregnancy overwith soon.

I had lost my mucous plug the day before and had begun to be excited, but one of my midwives said, "Well, you know, it could easily be two more weeks, so don't get too anxious."

Connie, an old high school friend, was visiting from New York City. She had not been invited to be a birth attendant, but she happened to be here and I am really glad things worked out that way. James, my husband, had gone to work in another town. Connie and I did several loads of wash and other chores.

I got more and more uncomfortable, was unable to find a comfortable position or take a nap. I bathed several more times; it was a warm day. I urinated every 15 minutes, it seemed, and had diarrhea most of the day. I was not perceiving the contractions as waves with a beginning and an ending. Once in a while I had to stop and sit down when I felt particularly uncomfortable.

I was sitting on the bed—we were waiting for James to get home—it was getting to be later-than-usual return time, and I had been feeling more and more uncomfortable. I had rocked up onto my hands and knees because of the tension in my abdomen, and Connie was rubbing my back a little when . . . gush! There was warm water all over my legs, and we knew this was it. Connie called the midwives who had to come from three other towns, and tried to reach Jim at work. His boss said he and his brother, Brion, had left a long time ago, so she called a friend and found Brion, who said he would bring Jim. It turned out James had been walking the several miles home because he wanted the chance to be alone and gather himself for the forthcoming event. When Jim arrived, I had cleaned up and changed and was sitting in the rocker shaking some. Connie was making the bed with a rubber sheet and fresh "sterile" sheets. Jim kissed me, and I told him, "Yep, I guess it's happening." Russ, one midwife, arrived at about 7:00 P.M. After greetings, he unpacked his satchel, took my blood pressure, and started timing contractions. He brought a confidence and a calming influence in with him.

The contractions were getting stronger, and I gradually stopped talking. I had moved to the bed. James stayed close to me the whole time; holding me, making suggestions, and being a very great comfort. I felt best sitting cross-legged or in the Zen Sitting Position and just breathing—letting these indescribable sensations wash over me. The other midwives arrived and wanted to examine me, but they had to wait for me to be able to lie back. One of them thought she heard two heartbeats and there was a lot of water with each contraction, so there was a hurried phone call to a consulting registered nurse-midwife to ask how to know if it really was twins. This was a rough time during the labor. I am sure I looked very self absorbed, but I certainly heard every word that was said. Finally I said, "So what if it is twins? I'll just push them both out and . . ." "No, if it is twins, you have to go to the hospital—not because the delivery is necessarily tricky, but because one of them might be small, weak, and really in need of hospital care." I was beginning to grunt, feeling the urge to push, and Russ and James were helping me pant. My blood pressure was checked again, and it had gone way up. Finally Joan checked me and found that I was completely dilated and that the head, which was way down, was a good-sized one, signalling a single birth. I was told that I could push and that we were not going to rush off to any hospital. Thank God.

Pushing was hard, hard work. I didn't have my act together for the first few pushes: I was puffing out my cheeks instead of holding my breath down low. After a while I got the hang of it. I rested, and then felt the contraction build. I pushed hard right in the middle of it and then rested again. I also kept changing my position, first pushing on my hands and knees, then squatting, then half sitting, half lying back, then back to squatting, and finally, back to hands and knees. A week later, Russ told me something interesting he had noticed during that part of the labor. As the progress of each push would gradually decrease, I would change my position, and on the next push there would be a marked improvement in the progress of the baby. I tried wiggling my hips on some of the heaviest pushes, and I believe it helped. That feeling of the baby sliding back in after a push was so frustrating—it felt like one step forward, two steps back—but I knew that the baby was getting closer and closer. I kept up an internal talk with the baby. This is something we did in the yoga class which I particularly appreciated. Midwives, my husband, and my friend were encouraging me at every push, and I was encouraging the baby. The baby was giving me back those moments of blessed peace in the midst of the greatest turmoil my body has ever experienced.

Before the pushing, when the contractions were peaking and it was all I could do to breathe and deal with them, I had the strangest sensation that the top of my being was about a foot and a half higher than the top of my head. I am sure that I could have felt that higher top with my hands if I had only been capable of moving my body.

I also should mention that the sensations of birth were such that I could have easily screamed and struggled, but I felt at the time (thanks to preparation, support, and grace) that it would hurt more if I had tightened up and screamed. So I sat and rocked a little and moaned. I made an "O" sound and visualized opening for the baby and I prayed. They were not long prayers—just little "ejaculations," I think they call them—"Mother of God, help me!" and so on.

I lost all sense of time as labor progressed. Just after midnight when the clock said I had been pushing for about an hour and a half and when it seemed that I could not hold my breath or push anymore, the head finally stretched me open that little bit more, then popped out and turned instead of slipping back. I said, "Oh, Thank God," and James told me Jason had his eyes open and was looking straight at him. I rested and heard the midwives beginning to suction the baby and counsel James on how to "catch" him as the rest of him came out. Another push or two for the shoulders and then . . . whoosh, a baby! Now I was still up on my hands and knees, so I was not seeing much, but I was listening to the little mewing noise that the new little one made and I was hearing the midwives and James and Connie all exclaiming about *him*—a boy, just as I had thought. I stayed up on my knees and rested a bit. His cord was so short that as soon as he was out he was tugging on his placenta, so they clamped and cut his cord right away and suctioned him some more. Someone helped me sit back without sitting on the clamp at my end of the cord. I held our new baby and said, "Hi there, you little guster." Everyone left James and me and the new one alone together—they went out to look at the stars and we just sat in bed and looked in each other's eyes. (The baby's were much more open than mine were. My face was badly swollen for almost a week after the birth because of "subcutaneous emphysema," which means that there was a little hole in my lung and air was forced up into the tissues of my shoulders, neck and face and was trapped there. I think this resulted from overpushing. Instead of following my own urges, I responded to the cheerleading of a zealous midwife.)

I felt another contraction or two and wanted to push out the placenta, so the midwives came in and someone got a pan and in no time and little effort, the placenta was out, too. James was holding the baby. Jason was a beautiful, skinny, curled-up little peaceful being with large hands and feet, weighing about seven and a half pounds. He snuggled on top of my belly instead of inside it.

Everything changed so fast those days. Our conditions, individually and as a family, were completely transformed. Jason came from inside, where it was warm, dark, and wet, to a world of air, light, people, milk, meconium, and urine. I went from big belly to empty belly and full breasts and arms. I had a swollen face, skinny legs, a happy heart and a new perspective on the cosmos. James went from one bedfellow to two, from being just a husband to a father as well. We kept looking at each other with tears in our eyes those days—tears of awe, gratitude, union.

Author's note: Many home birth supplies can be obtained from Cascade Birthing Supplies Center. The address is 718 SW 16th Street, Corvallis, OR, 97330.

HOSPITAL BIRTH

This is Naomi and David Howe's birth story. You might like to know that Naomi is the model in this book. She and David are pictured as well in chapter 11 on massage. You can see Dana, their first child, in the Appendix.

In keeping with my daily outdoor excursions, Dave and I decided to go to a nearby park because it was such a beautiful February day. We walked along the river for a while enjoying the sun and water but had to come back early because the wind was quite strong. I was a little disappointed, so on the way home Dave suggested that we stop for some pizza at Spiro's restaurant. I love pizza—who was I to refuse? I squeezed into the booth and we indulged in a nice small plain pizza. I was feeling restless, somehow.

Later that afternoon, while Chinese brushpainting, I felt a little bit of water leak—or was it urine?—and went to the bathroom. I continued painting until mild menstrual-like cramps began with some regularity. Dave walked in, saw me staring into space and said, "What's the matter?" "Oh, nothing much," I replied, "except that I think today is the day!" After a few incredulous glances and smiles, we decided to go upstairs and shower. After our shower we got our things together to take to the hospital. Not too bad, I thought, if this is what labor is supposed to be!

My contractions seemed very much like strong menstrual cramps; they were not too regular but were beginning to come three to five minutes apart. I was having a slight bloody show, a little mucous, and the continuous water loss. Dave was marching around with watch in hand; I thought this was quite humorous.

At 5:30 P.M. I called the hospital to tell them about my water breaking and the progress of the contractions. I talked to Dr. Zwerner, one of my obstetricians, who said to come into the hospital. It finally hit me "This is really it—in a few hours I will have a baby!" We took our time, since I was still quite comfortable, and made sure to put our new baby seat in the car.

When we arrived at the hospital, we went to the Admitting Office and filled out all the forms. I was very proud of the fact that I was joking and talking to the secretary there in the office. I was feeling pretty good, although still leaking steadily. I had worn a super maxipad to the hospital, and it worked quite well. From there I was wheeled up to Labor and Delivery by Penny, the nurse who had showed us around that part of the hospital when we had our tour. Dave was right by me the entire time, which was a great comfort, since I was no expert at hospital procedure. Since no one else was in labor at the time, I was able to use the hospital's birthing room, and I was delighted. (In this room a woman may labor and give birth to her baby with the help and companionship of her husband or any other person she chooses.) Penny called Dr. Zwerner and he arrived a short time later. My blood pressure and temperature were checked, and a routine blood test was taken. I was not prepped, and had no monitor or I.V.

After Dr. Zwerner examined me, he said I was three centimeters dilated and in "early labor." He said he would return about 9:00 or 10:00 P.M. unless I was "setting the world on fire" before then. Penny mentioned that we could get up and walk around and that sounded like a great idea. I put on my robe & slippers, stuffed a blue pad into the pocket, and away we went. Dave was already in hospital greens since he would be with me all through the birthing process. We cruised the hospital halls, went down to the obstetrics office, up to the intensive care unit, through Maternity, to the T.V. room, and so on. After a while the hospital walls became pretty routine and we began to run out of jokes! Dave was keeping a close monitor with his official timing device! We called both sets of parents to let them know what the story was. My mother-in-law's birthday was the next day, so she was hoping for a midnight delivery! Just not too much beyond that, I hoped!

By 9:00 P.M., my contractions were becoming difficult to cope with; I was close to crumpling in the hallway! They were two to three minutes apart and sometimes one and a half to two minutes long. So we limped our way back to the birthing room. Penny had been searching us out every hour or so, checking the baby's heartbeat which was 148 and steady. When we returned, she checked my blood pressure again, and all seemed to be fine. I was still working with the Early Labor breath, which worked well with the contractions. I sat on the bed in a yoga cross-legged position as well as various other sitting positions. I found laboring on my hands and knees with a pillow placed on the edge of the bed which I could use as a headrest often effective, although nothing was truly comfortable. I found that I could not put weight on my bottom during contractions or it increased the sensations. Often I pushed on the bed with my hands to raise my body (which was in a cross-legged position) during a contraction. This was tiring for my arms, but it eased the discomfort of the contraction so that I could breathe through it. I kept my eyes on Dave's eyes as the breathing became more difficult. Aha, I thought, so *this* is active labor. Not something to schedule on your day off, Naomi! Dr. Zwerner came back to check me and found I was 5 centimeters dilated and the cervix was paper thin. He indicated that the thinning would facilitate dilation. I continued to breathe through contractions at this point using Who-Who-Ha breaths as Dave called out 3 and 1, or 2 and 1, or 1 and 1 variations of the breath.

At 11:00 P.M. I was still in transition although I did not experience the feelings I had heard about such as irrationality and irritability. I did, however, throw Dave scathing glances whenever he said "Relax!" Occasionally I let out small cries particulary at the beginning of a contraction as I struggled to maintain control. This was partly because in between contractions or during rest periods I often would actually fall asleep on Dave's shoulder! I had little difficulty relaxing between contractions, although the power of the contractions made it quite difficult at times to maintain controlled breathing. A great benefit was the focal point of Dave's eyes. I really thought of his eyes as my lifeline to reality!

At midnight Dr. Zwerner said I could push because I was finally fully dilated. I had some trouble finding a comfortable pushing position and was not really prepared to push. My back arched due to the flatness of the bed. Even with a wedge, I couldn't find a really effective pushing position. I was getting tired from the pushing, and the baby wasn't making much progress down the birth canal. However, I *was* able to completely relax and fall asleep between contractions, and this helped to conserve my strength. The time went by fast, each contraction forced me into the "here and now!"

By 1:30 A.M., I had made little progress, but I could feel the baby move down a little more. I was feeling discouraged that I was still pushing, but Dave was, as always, optimistic and smiling, helping me on.

Dr. Zwerner examined me, and then used a surgical hook to break my waters completely. From that time on I could really see my abdominal muscles move and feel the baby head on out. Dave was really excited, and kept me posted "I can see the head!" The pushing was much easier and felt terrific. Finally the baby's head stayed crowned and did not move back up the canal!

Dr. Zwerner sat on the end of the bed and gave me novocaine for an episiotomy. There was absolutely no pain. The pushes seemed easier now because I knew the birth was near. He did three episiotomy clips with scissors (I felt only pressure) and helped the baby to ease out by pressing his fingers against my rectum, which was an extremely uncomfortable sensation, to say the least. He had me turn on my side at this time and he helped the head out. I cried out, but *what* a relief! I was elated; Dave was ready and waiting with camera, and then we saw him!

At 2:17 A.M., Dana Christopher Howe arrived in the world! "Well, it's about time, Dana Christopher," were my first words to him. He was cleaned up with a few wipes, wrapped in a blanket, and put on my stomach. What a beautiful boy!

After the placenta was born, about five minutes later, Dr. Zwerner stitched my episiotomy, and then left us all alone for the next hour. I felt a great sense of relief that the physical aspect of the birth was over and was delighted to see my baby. My tiredness miraculously vanished. I tried to nurse him there on the table, but he was not very interested. I thought, "This is no candidate for Overeaters Anonymous." Dave was ecstatic about the baby and picked him up soon after birth, at which point Dana immediately stopped crying. We looked at him, babbled at him, and admired Dana until 3:30 A.M., when Dave decided to call his parents and mine. They even wheeled me out in the hall (on a table) to talk to them as well. I was a little weak, but, after all—it was Mom's birthday too! Then we called my folks—of course, all were delighted. True to form, my Mom and Dad broke out some champagne at 4:00 A.M. to celebrate!

CESAREAN SECTION BIRTH

At the present time many hospitals have instituted new rules allowing husbands to accompany their wives into the delivery room for a planned or low-risk Cesarean birth. One young couple, Michael and Betty Ann Conroy, who had had a difficult history with prior births, describe their very rewarding C-section experience.

Michael's Story

When my wife, Betty Ann, first told me about the "Yoga for the Mother-to-Be" classes, I was not very interested and doubtful of the benefits. The main reason I was skeptical was that we knew that she would have to have a C-section and could see no benefit from toning muscles that are used for natural childbirth. My wife's past medical history was also very discouraging. Ten weeks after we were married, she had major surgery to remove a tumor the size of a grapefruit from her uterus. After this operation her doctors were concerned about how her uterus would bear up, if she were to become pregnant. We decided to take the risk, but unfortunately Betty Ann's first pregnancy ended at 6 months with the loss of a set of twin girls. Even after this heartbreaking experience, Betty Ann and I were determined to have a baby. The second pregnancy ended happily with the birth via C-section of a healthy, beautiful 9 lb. 4 oz. baby boy, whom we named Michael. Although this was a successful pregnancy, the months that Betty Ann carried were full of hard times. She spent a good deal of time in bed and had to stay flat on her back for the last four months because of high blood pressure.

As Michael was growing up, we decided that we would be happy having a second child. However, the third pregnancy ended in a miscarriage after the third month. The three pregnancies had taken their toll on Betty Ann's uterus, for it had become very weak and paper thin. As with Michael's birth, a C-section was a necessity: the pressure on her uterus during labor was expected to burst it, resulting in disaster for both her and the baby.

Betty Ann and I entered the fourth pregnancy haunted by the past. I was hoping for the best, but I was preparing myself for the worst. My wife was in her second month when she first started her yoga classes. She was very excited when she got home from her first class. She eagerly tried to explain what the benefits of the exercises were. However, I still was not convinced that they would benefit Betty Ann, since she was not going to be able to have a normal delivery.

It was in her fifth month when I suddenly realized how well her pregnancy was going. She was attending weekly classes and practicing her exercises and deep breathing faithfully. She looked and felt good and was not bothered by nagging backaches, which she had experienced with Michael's pregnancy. I was invited to attend yoga class with her one night, and I did all the exercises she had been doing. I also learned how to give my wife a massage to relax her and make her feel better. Better yet, she gave me one as well! It was at this time that I really started to feel I was an important part of her pregnancy. The months seemed to go by much faster than before. We stopped worrying about possible problems and complications, which allowed us to relax and enjoy the later months.

The doctor had set a date for the C-section one week before Betty Ann's due date. She and I were sure that she would not make it to the C-section date, because Michael had been two weeks early. Betty Ann did make it on time, and we had a 9 lb. 9½ oz., 21½ inch long baby girl, whom we named Tammy Ann. I was present in the delivery room while Betty received partial anesthesia and then had a C-section. I was even able to take color photos of the event as it was happening. The medical team worked quickly and efficiently, for very soon after the incisions were made, my baby daughter was born. There were no problems late in the pregnancy as had happened previously. Betty Ann was even able to attend a bowling banquet, a wedding reception and a graduation party, all within the last four days before her C-section. How different from the last successful pregnancy, when she had to spend the last four months in bed.

I really believe that attending the yoga classes and learning to relax played a very vital role in making this pregnancy go so well for us.

Betty Ann's Story

I was admitted to the hospital the night before my scheduled C-section, where I was watched all night because I was having some mild contractions. At five A.M. the nurses began preparing me for the operation. I had to have an enema and an IV inserted, as well as a catheter, to drain my urine. None of these procedures was painful. Then at eight A.M. I was wheeled on a table into the delivery room to be anesthetized for the C-section. The most difficult part for me was trying to be perfectly still during the injection of the spinal anesthesia. I concentrated on my yogic deep breathing and completely relaxing. The medical staff said that I relaxed very well. It took a while for the anesthesia to numb the bottom part of my body, but by 8:25 A.M. my baby girl was born.

It was beautiful. Mike was so excited and I was totally speechless!

Mike kept yelling, "It's a girl! It's a girl, Betty!" After the doctors lifted her out of my abdomen, they put a tube in her mouth to suction her and make it easier for her to breathe. Then they put her in a blanket and handed her to Mike and me. I could not take my eyes off her as Mike held her. Hearing our baby cry out for the first time while her father was holding her was, to me, the most beautiful experience of all. Soon the doctors took her from Mike and put her on my chest. One of my arms was attached to a blood pressure gauge while the other one had IV tubes in it, so I was not able to hold her, but I could look at her while she lay on my chest, all warm and new. Mike was right next to me and held her steady on my chest. I just kept kissing and talking to her. She was crying and so was I!

Even though I had a C-section, I had a very positive and meaningful bonding experience with my daughter. While they were sewing up my incision, Tammy remained on my chest or in Mike's arms. I really felt overjoyed to have my husband experience the birth and the bonding time during Tammy Ann's birth.

After a short while Tammy was taken to the nursery to be weighed and cleaned up. A few hours later, when I was returned to my room, the nurses brought Tammy back to see us.

I had to remain flat on my back for the 12 hours following my daughter's birth due to the anesthesia. However, the deep breathing helped a great deal during that time. I was up and about 13 hours after Tammy was born. My stitched area was sore, but I felt really good and was able to walk around for a while.

I have had three other pregnancies and none have been nearly as terrific as this one was. I know it was because I kept practicing my yoga exercises. The exercises especially helped during my recovery period. I had Tammy on Wednesday morning and I went home on Sunday morning. My daughter is nursing well, and I feel good because I did my nipple preparation.

I cannot truly express in words how much help I received from my yoga training. It is a wonderful system for pregnant women, their husbands and, of course, their babies!

A FINAL NOTE

The birth of your baby can be a very high, exciting, and joyous experience. The three weeks following the birth are often a time of adjustment and fatigue. The following tips should be quite helpful to you:

- Try to have someone to help you (full time, if possible) during the first one to two weeks postpartum. This will enable you to rest and recuperate more quickly.
- Rest or sleep as much as you can at this time.
- Relieve engorged breasts by using a breast pump or by taking a hot shower.
- Keep taking your prenatal vitamins with iron.
- Eat four to six small nutritious meals a day.
- Snack and drink liquids often.
- Do Yogic Abdominal Breathing to relax so that you can easily feed your baby.
- Have faith in yourself and your parenting abilities.

When you are living through the birthday of your child, you think you will always remember every detail, but often the experience fades from memory. I strongly recommend that you write down in detail all the events of this very important day in your life. It is fun in later years to go back and mentally relive this very exciting day.

I wish you a positive and enjoyable pregnancy and birth experience. Good luck and have fun with your new parenting role. I am truly happy to have shared this prenatal yoga program with you. I wish you joy, fulfillment, and om shanti, peace.

Appendix

MEET THE MODELS

I have indeed been fortunate to work with very special people while preparing the photographic illustrations for this book. Since you will be constantly looking at these models, while you learn to do the various postures, I thought that you might want to know a bit about their lives and interests. Let me introduce them to you.

Naomi, David and Dana Howe

Naomi and Dave are the couple who have been featured throughout this book. They live in Connecticut with their dog, Sebastian, their cat, Nicholas, and of course the newest member of their family, Dana Christopher. In 1974, Naomi graduated from Connecticut College with a degree in Asian Studies and psychology while Dave attended Lehigh University where he graduated in 1973 with a degree in Industrial Engineering and Arts. Both of them love to sing and play music. Dave plays the guitar, piano and organ, and Naomi is a violinist with the Eastern Connecticut Symphony Orchestra (Fig. AP–1). Naomi's other activities include teaching yoga classes, acting as chairman of her town's planning commission as well as being a member of the Phenix Club (a senior citizens meditation and discussion group) and a weekly meditation group. In those few spare moments during the week, she studies T'ai Chi and Chinese brush painting. Dave is a computer enthusiast extraordinaire (AP–2), but takes time to go skiing, skating, hiking, and sailing with his wife and son. Mostly they have a great time enjoying the circle of life and sharing it with their new son.

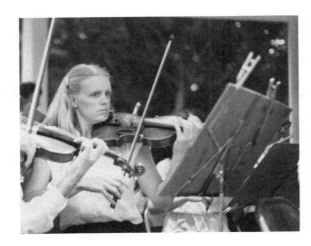

Figure AP.1 Naomi playing the violin with the Eastern Connecticut Symphony Orchestra.

Figure AP.2 David and Dana enjoying the computer.

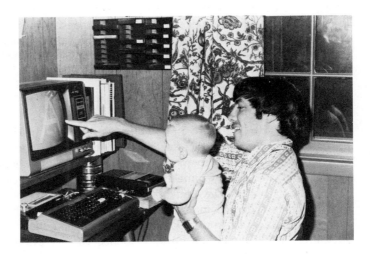

LIST OF AVAILABLE PRACTICE CASSETTE TAPES

In order to help my students develop the correct timing and sequence for practicing, I have always made 60 minute cassette practice tapes available. I have personally recorded a set of tapes which can be easily utilized in conjunction with this book. The tapes contain two 30 minute sequences based on the yogic program which has been presented in this book.

The following tapes are available:

Tape 1

Side One:
- Yogic Breathing Techniques
- The Salute to the Child
- Complete Relaxation

Side Two:
- The Basic 9
- Pelvic Floor Exercises

Tape 2

Side One:

- Yogic Breathing and "Inner Bonding Techniques"
- Standing and Sitting Asanas
- Pelvic Floor Exercises

Side Two:

- Breathing for Birth

Additional tapes on stress management postpartum shape up with baby exercises, massage, and varied breathing and meditational techniques are also available.

To obtain a current price list, send a self-addressed envelope to:

BE HEALTHY TAPES c/o Sylvia Klein Olkin, 4 Lauren Lane, Norwich, Ct. 06360.

- Please allow 6 weeks for delivery.
- If you have personal queries, you can write to me using the above address. I would be happy to hear from you.

PRACTICE SCHEDULES

During Pregnancy

You should practice the following exercises 20–30 minutes *every* day or *every* other day:

1. Rock-the-Baby breath
2. The Basic Nine or
3. The Salute to the Child
4. Complete Relaxation with Concentration or Meditation
5. Any other pregnancy asanas you desire

During the Last Six Weeks of Pregnancy

You should practice the following exercises for 20–30 minutes, preferably with your coach.

1. Breathing for Birth breaths; 10–15 minute practice session; practice each breath so that you can comfortably do it for 60–90 seconds.
2. Complete Relaxation
3. Various positions for labor and birth; hold each position 1–3 minutes.
4. The Salute to the Child
5. The Pregnancy Sit-up (number 6 of the Basic Nine)
6. Any other pregnancy asanas you desire

During the First Three Weeks Postpartum

You should practice the following exercises beginning immediately after the baby's birth. Try to practice some of them while you take care of the baby.

Exercises After a Vaginal Delivery:

1. Pelvic Floor exercises; begin these right after the baby's birth. Do 300 per day while feeding the baby, resting, watching television, etc.
2. Yogic Abdominal breath with retention: inhale through your nose into your abdomen; exhale through your nose while trying to pull the abdomen in. Don't breathe as you try to hold the tummy in. Inhale and repeat. Do 15–20 times a day while feeding the baby, resting, etc.
3. Complete relaxation lying on your tummy: place a pillow under your head and another one under your abdomen. Relax fully for 15–20 minutes in this position.
4. Anal lock in the shower to quickly heal postpartum hemorrhoids. See pp. 92–94 for full instructions.
5. Pregnancy Sit-Up, number six of the Basic Nine, repeat three times.
6. Pregnancy Spinal Twist, number three of the Basic Nine, repeat three times.
7. Single Leg Lifts: lying flat on your back take 10 seconds to lift one leg straight up into the air. Hold it up 10 seconds. Slowly lower it to the mat taking 15–20 seconds. Take 1–2 deep breaths. Repeat on other side. Do three more times. After two weeks, do double leg lifts by placing your hands palms down under your lower back and lifting both legs up into the air.

8. Head to Knee Pose: lying flat on your back, lift one leg straight up. Bend the leg onto your chest and wrap your arms around the knee. Bring your forehead to your knee and hold 30 seconds to two minutes. Lower the head, release the arms, straighten and lower the leg slowly, using the abdominal muscles. Repeat on other side. Do three more times.

Exercises after a Cesarean Birth:

1. Exercises 1–4, as listed under "Exercises after a Vaginal Delivery," can be practiced during the first two to three weeks.

2. The Bridge with Preparatory Pelvic Rocking, number four of the Basic Nine, can be practiced beginning the third week postpartum.

3. The Pregnancy Sit-Up, number six of the Basic Nine, can be practiced during the third week postpartum.

After 21–28 days your abdominal muscle tone will return and you can resume a regular yoga program. Try to practice yoga with your baby every day. Happy practicing!

Glossary

ANAL MUSCLES. Muscles which open and close the rectal outlet.

ANEMIA. A condition in which the red corpuscles of the blood are reduced in number or are deficient in hemoglobin.

ANUS. Muscular outlet of the rectum which is the lower end of the large intestine.

ASANA. Yoga postures, poses, or movements. Literally translated from Sanskrit, it means easy, firm, steady position.

BABY BREATH. A special breathing technique which facilitates inner bonding and helps to prepare for the pushing stage of labor.

BIRTH CANAL. The vagina, through which the baby passes in order to be born.

BIRTH MANDALA. A geometric design which has been especially created for you to use as an outward focus during labor and delivery (see also MANDALA).

BLOODY SHOW. The mucous plug (often tinged with blood) which is released from the cervix before or during early labor.

BRAXTON-HICKS CONTRACTIONS. Physical contractions of the uterus all during pregnancy, which prepare the uterus for labor.

CERVIX. The lowest, bottleneck-shaped portion of the uterus which opens into the vagina or birth canal.

CESAREAN BIRTH. Birth of a baby using surgical incisions either in the abdominal or pubic area.

CHAKRA. (Pronounced chuk-ruh) Sanskrit word meaning internal energy center of the body. There are 7 energy centers, according to yogic theory.

COLOSTRUM. The first fluid secreted by the mother's breasts before her milk comes in. It is high in antibodies and protein.

CONTRACTION. A tensing or shortening of the muscle fibers of the uterus, which is followed by a relaxation or lengthening of these fibers.

CROWNING. Visual appearance of the baby's head at the vaginal or birth canal outlet.

DIAPHRAGM. A large, thick muscle which separates the chest (thorax) from the abdomen. This is the muscle which is used in Yogic Abdominal ("Rock-the-Baby") Breath.

DILATATION. The stretching open of the cervix during the first stage of labor. Always measured in centimeters.

EDEMA. Bodily swelling caused by excess fluid retained in the body's tissues.

EFFACEMENT. Thinning of the cervix prior or during labor.

EPISIOTOMY. Surgical incision or cut, usually made with scissors, of the perineum (outer birth canal) to give the baby's head more room, prevent tearing of the vagina, and make the birth smoother.

FETUS. Medical term for the baby as it grows inside from the third month to the end of the pregnancy.

HATHA YOGA. (Pronounced Huh-tuh yo-ga) A scientific physical system containing stretches, massage movements, breathing techniques, and relaxation practices, which leads to control of the physical body and vitality.

HEMORRHOIDS. Inflamed and often painful veins of the rectum.

IN UTERO. Within the uterus.

INTRAVENOUS INFUSION (IV). Fluids or medication administered through the vein via a needle and drip bottle.

KUNDALINI ENERGY. (Pronounced Koon-dah-lee-nee) A Sanskrit term for latent spiritual force or inner energy.

LACTATION. The secretion or formation of milk, or the period of milk production in the female body.

LIGHTENING. Descent of the baby into the pelvis.

LOCHIA. Vaginal discharge after delivery.

MANDALA. (Pronounced Mun-dah'-luh) The Sanskrit word for circle or center. It consists of a series of concentric forms. In many cultures the mandala has symbolized the entire cosmos and the dot placed within it, the essence or the source of things. It is used for centering and concentrating.

MANTRAS. (Pronounced Muhn-truh) The sacred words and sounds which have been used in Eastern countries for centuries for healing and spiritual development.

MEDITATION. The relaxation of the body and the quieting of the mind during concentration on the breath, or an internal or external sound.

MIDWIFE. A person who assists women in childbirth.

MISCARRIAGE. Loss of the baby before the end of the seventh month of pregnancy.

OM. (Pronounced Ohm) The highest mantra; the vibration of life energy.

PELVIC FLOOR. Muscle layers which form a sling across the base of the pelvis and support the bladder, uterus, and rectum.

PELVIS. The bones which form the two hip bones, the sacrum, and the tailbone.

PERINEUM. The area between the anus and the external genitals.

PLACENTA. An organ which nourishes the unborn child via the umbilical cord all during the pregnancy. After the baby is born, the placenta is born and called the afterbirth.

POSTPARTUM. The period of time, following the birth of the baby, before the mother returns to her prepregnancy condition.

PRANA. (Pronounced Prah-nuh) The Sanskrit word for breath. The absolute energy or life-giving force which pervades the universe and all who live therein.

PRANAYAMAS. (Pronounced Prah-nah-yah-muh) Breathing exercises for strengthening the lungs, calming down, or energizing, with strong emphasis on repetitive inhalations and exhalations.

PRENATAL. The time period during pregnancy before the baby is born.

QUICKENING. The first movements of the fetus felt by the mother. Usually this occurs between the sixteenth and twentieth weeks of growth.

RAJA YOGA. (Pronounced Rah-jyuh) Literally, the royal path, or the study of meditation.

"ROCK-THE-BABY" BREATH. Yogic Abdominal Breathing to be used during all the pregnancy months.

ROOT CHAKRA. First basic energy center of the body located between the anus and the genital area.

ROUND LIGAMENTS. Fibrous muscle connecting the uterus and the pelvic bones.

SUPINE POSITION. Postures which begin while lying flat on the back.

UMBILICAL CORD. The physical connection which supplies the unborn baby with its nourishment. It contains two arteries and one vein to carry oxygen, nutrients, and waste products between the placenta and the baby.

URETHRA. The narrow passageway through which urine is discharged from the bladder.

UTERUS. The womb in which the baby grows during the nine months of pregnancy.

VAGINA. The muscular birth canal leading from the uterus to the outer genitals.

VARICOSE VEINS. Swollen, painful veins, usually of the legs, but often in the genitals, too.

YIN AND YANG. In Chinese thought, the complementary forces pervading the universe. The interactions of these two forces cause things to happen.

YOGA. (Pronounced Yo-guh) A Sanskrit word meaning "to yoke or fasten together." A scientific system for bringing about a natural balance in the mind, the body, and the spirit.

Bibliography

Breastfeeding

LA LECHE LEAGUE INTERNATIONAL. *The Womanly Art of Breastfeeding,* 1963.
A very thorough guide to breastfeeding by the organization which has been counseling nursing women for over 20 years. Good factual information. Very conventional attitudes about the role of women.

PRYOR, KAREN. *Nursing Your Baby,* 1973.
Well written guide for new nursing mothers.

Cesarean Birth

CESAREAN INFORMATION GROUP. *Frankly Speaking, a Pamphlet for Cesarean Couples,* 49 Top Stone Drive; Danbury, CT 06801. Fee: $3.00.

DONOVAN, BONNIE. *The Cesarean Birth Experience: a Practical, Comprehensive and Reassuring Guide for Parents and Professionals,* 1977.
A very thorough guide for women who know they will be having a Cesarean birth and for those who want to be prepared. Covers pregnancy, birth, and postpartum. Highly recommended.

MEYER, LINDA. *The Cesarean Revolution: a Handbook for Parents and Childbirth Educators,* 1979.
The options available for Cesarean couples are discussed.

Childbirth

BING, ELIZABETH. *Six Practical Lessons for an Easier Childbirth,* 1977.
A step-by-step Lamaze guide by a well known childbirth educator. Standard reading when taking Lamaze classes.

DICK-READ, GRANTLY. *Childbirth without Fear,* 1972.
A wonderful book by the originator of prepared childbirth. Contains a good discussion on the relationship between relaxation and easier labor and birth. Recommended.

FELDMAN, SYLVIA. *Choices in Childbirth,* 1978.
A thorough, well-organized, and practical approach to the alternatives in childbirth. Includes sections on hospital birth and home birth with a midwife. A good book with basic information.

FENLON, ARLENE; MCPHERSON, ELLEN; and DORCHAK, LOVELL. *Getting Ready for Childbirth,* 1979.
An excellent guidebook on all aspects of pregnancy and birth. Some information on pastpartum is provided as well. Highly recommended.

GOLD, E. J., DR.; and GOLD, CYBELE, DR. *Joyous Childbirth,* 1977.
A manual for conscious natural childbirth delving deeply into the natural birth approach. Some information is practical, some highly psychological.

INTERNATIONAL CHILDBIRTH EDUCATION ASSOCIATION. Bookcenter, Box 20048, 8060 26th Ave. So.; Minneapolis, MN 55420.
Most of the books concerning pregnancy, birth, and parenting can be ordered through the ICEA. Write to the ICEA to have your name added to their mailing list.

KITZINGER, SHEILA. *Experience of Childbirth,* 1972.
A top-notch book on the many aspects of pregnancy and birth written by a famous British childbirth educator. Takes the human aspect into account. Highly recommended.

KITZINGER, SHEILA. *Giving Birth,* 1977.
A variety of personal birth stories dealing with the parents' emotions in childbirth. If you like to read birth stories, this book is for you.

LEBOYER, FREDERICK. *Birth Without Violence,* 1975.
A book about a quiet, peaceful, respectful birth for your baby using the Leboyer method of quiet and birth bath. Beautifully written and illustrated with sensitive photos. Highly recommended.

MILINARE, CATERINE. *Birth: Facts and Legends,* 1971.
An artistic and joyful book, beautifully illustrated with drawings, photos, and diagrams about the experience of childbirth. Recommended.

Cookbooks

ELLIOT, SHARON; and HAIGHT, SANDY. *The Busy People's Naturally Delicious Decidedly Delicious Fast Food Book,* 1977.
Quick and natural fast food snacks. Many are high in calories, but some are tasty and nutritious. Contains some tasty, quick, and nutritious refrigerator recipes.

FORD, MARJORIE; HILLYARD, SUSAN; and KOOCK, MARY FAULK. *The Deaf Smith Country Cookbook,* 1973.
A variety of vegetarian recipes, many from the southwest of the U.S. Good section on snacks and sandwiches as well as very tasty soups.

HEWITT, JEAN. *The New York Times Natural Foods Cookbook,* 1972.
Hundreds of recipes using natural ingredients. Has a good section on homemade baby food.

KATZEN, MOLLIE. *Moosewood Cookbook,* 1977.
A beautifully illustrated, creative vegetarian cookbook based on the recipes used in the Moosewood Restaurant. The variety and ingenuity plus tastiness of the recipes makes this book a must to own if you want to learn more about vegetarian cooking. Highly recommended.

LAPPE, FRANCES MOORE. *Diet for Small Planet,* 1973.
The source book on complementary proteins. An excellent discussion of how incomplete proteins can be combined to make high-grade protein nutrition. Also contains a variety of recipes to put the ideas into practice.

ROBERTSON, LAUREL; FLINDERS, CAROL; and GODFREY, BRONWEN. *Laurel's Kitchen,* 1978.
A complete reference book for vegetarian cooking. Has a huge variety of recipes plus a folksy manner and thorough nutritional charts. Highly recommended.

Exercise

BALASKAS, ARTHUR; and BALASKAS, JANET. *New Life: The Book of Exercises for Childbirth,* London, 1979.
This beautiful, creative, and highly educational book presents the British viewpoint of prepared childbirth. Highly recommended.

NOBLE, ELISABETH. *Essential Exercises for the Childbearing Year,* 1976.
Well-explained exercises and extensive text on pregnancy and postpartum. Includes rehabilitation after a C-Section. Nicely illustrated with line drawings. Recommended.

Hatha Yoga

ARYA, USHARBUDH. *Philosophy of Hatha Yoga,* Himalayan International Institute of Yoga Science and Philosophy of USA, 1977.
Integrates the philosophy of yogic practice with the physical aspects of yoga. Well written and practical.

FOLAN, LILIAS M. *Lilias, Yoga and You,* 1972.
A well illustrated guide to beginning Hatha Yoga by television Yoga Teacher, Lilias.

NEUMAN, DIANE. *How to Get the Dragons Out of Your Temple,* Celestial Arts, 1976.
A delightful hand written and illustrated book on physical yoga. Contains some very helpful pointers. Highly recommended.

PHELAN, NANCY; and VOLIN, MICHAEL. *Sex and Yoga,* 1967.
How yoga affects the sexual functioning of the body. It has a thorough discussion of tantra. Some photos and illustrations are included, but often directions for poses are not clear.

PHELAN, NANCY; and VOLIN, MICHAEL. *Yoga for Women,* 1963.
An interesting book written by two Australian yoga teachers. Often the directions for the asanas are not clear. There are some photos and some illustrations.

SAMSKRITI and VEDA. *Hatha Yoga, Manual One,* Himilayanian International Institute of Yoga Sciences and Philosophy, 1979.
An excellent beginner asana book. Well-illustrated but the benefits of each posture are not given.

SARASWATI, SWAMI MUKTANANDA. *Nawa Yogini Tantra,* Bihar School of Yoga, Monghyr, India, 1977.
A hatha yoga book written by a woman especially for women. Line drawings illustrate a variety of postures. Thorough discussion of meditation is included as well.

SATCHIDANANDA, SWAMI. *Integral Yoga Hatha,* 1970.
A very thorough and informative book on the various aspects of hatha yoga. Has some very interesting and challenging advanced postures.

ZEBROFF, KAREEN. *The ABC of Yoga,* Arco, 1979.
A well illustrated, organized and informative book for beginning yoga students. Well illustrated with numerous photos. Highly recommended.

ZEBROFF, KAREEN. *Yoga and Nutrition,* Arco, 1979.
An excellent, photographically-illustrated intermediate to advanced hatha yoga book. Discussion on nutrition is limited but interesting.

Health

BERKELLEY HOLISTIC HEALTH CENTER. *The Holistic Health Handbook,* 1978.
A source book of the many approaches to health. Includes articles on Oriental systems, native American systems, Western systems as well as techniques and practices of holistic health. A good reference book on the newest approaches to total health.

BOSTON'S HEALTH BOOK COLLECTIVE. *Our Bodies, Our Selves,* 1976.
An excellent book written by women to help other women understand themselves better. Contains an excellent chapter on childbirth. A very good source book.

KAPIT, WYNN; and ELSON, LAWRENCE M. *The Anatomy Coloring Book,* 1977.
Learn about the inner workings of your body by coloring each section. A fun book to work on as you learn.

SAMUELS, MIKE, M.D.; and BENNETT, HAL. *The Well Body Book,* 1975.
How to use the healing energy that your body possesses. A very good source book for learning more about how your body works or breaks down. Recommended.

Herbs

HYLTON, WILLIAM H., ed. *The Rodale Herb Book: How to Use, Grow, and Buy Nature's Miracle Plants,* 1978.
A source book on herbs and their uses.

MESSÉGUÉ, MAURICE. *Health Secrets of Plants and Herbs,* 1979.
A thorough discussion of the characteristics, contents and uses of many, many herbs.

MILLSPAUGH, CHARLES F. *American Medicinal Plants,* 1974.
Contains characteristics and uses of a variety of American herbs.

THOMSON, ROBERT. *Natural Medicine,* 1978.
Contains specific herbal recommendations for labor and delivery as well as an account of the author's wife's use of herbs when their child was born.

Home Birth

LANG, RAVEN. *The Birth Book,* 1972.
A very personal book on home birth; well illustrated with photos.

SOUSA, MARION. *Childbirth at Home,* 1977.
A complete discussion of the pros and cons of home birth. Must reading for any couple considering home birth.

WHITE, GREGORY J., M.D. *Emergency Childbirth,* 1976.
A factual handbook for emergency birth situations. Well worth reading.

Massage

DOWNING, GEORGE. *The Massage Book,* 1972.
A good basic book on massage strokes and technique. Well illustrated.

LEBOYER, FREDERICK. *Loving Hands: The Traditional Indian Art of Baby Massage,* 1976.
Beautiful prose, photographs, and feelings pervade this instructive book on baby massage.

Meditation

MISHRA, RAMMURTI. *Yoga Sutras,* 1973.
A textbook of yoga psychology based on the writings of the yogi, Patanjali. It explores the relationship between the psyche, the physical universe, and all branches of science.

ORNSTEIN, ROBERT. *The Psychology of Consciousness,* 1972.
A scientific exploration of the functioning of the two hemispheres of the brain for a better understanding of consciousness.

PECK, ROBERT L. *American Meditation and Beginning Yoga,* 1976.
A clear, well written, scientific approach and explanation of Raja Yoga as well as altered states of consciousness. This book is only available from Personal Development Center, Box 251, Windham Center, CT., 06280.

RAM DASS. *The Journey of Awakening: a Meditator's Guidebook,* 1978.
This book contains information on meditation as well as a state by state listing of available meditation groups. It is a good source for those students wishing to find other meditators. Highly recommended.

Nutrition

BREWER, TOM; and BREWER, GAIL. *What Every Pregnant Woman Should Know: the Truth About Diets and Drugs in Pregnancy,* 1977.
Carefully explains the relationship between good nutrition and having a healthy baby and a positive pregnancy. Good discussion on toxemia.

CALIFORNIA DEPARTMENT OF HEALTH SERVICES. *Nutrition During Pregnancy and Lactation,* 714–744 P Street, Sacramento, CA 95814.
A research report on nutritional requirements of different ethnic groups. Has good daily intake guidelines.

GOLDBECK, NIKKI. *As You Eat So Your Baby Grows,* 1979.
This well illustrated pamphlet is must reading for all pregnant women.

Concisely explains what should be part of a balanced prenatal diet. It is available for $1.50 from: CERES PRESS, Box 87, Woodstock, NY 12498. Highly recommended.

GOLDBECK, NIKKI; and GOLDBECK, DAVID. *The Supermarket Handbook,* 1973.
A very handy book for learning what processed and natural foods really contain. Recommended.

JACOBSON, MICHAEL F. *Nutrition Scoreboard,* Revised, 1979.
An excellent book with a unique scoreboard system for learning the best foods for good health.

LANSKY, VICKI. *The Taming of the C.A.N.D.Y. Monster (Continuously Advertised Nutritionally Deficient Yummies),* 1977.
A guide for eliminating or minimizing your child's consumption of junk food. Has good ideas for high nutrition snacks, desserts, etc. Good for when children are preschool and school age.

NUTRITION SEARCH, INC. *Nutrition Almanac,* 1979.
A basic book on understanding nutrition. Has comprehensive charts on the vitamin, mineral, and caloric content of numerous foods. Recommended.

PELSTRING, LINDA; and HAVEN, JO-ANN. *Food to Improve Your Health,* 1974.
This book will tell you what is in your food nutritionally and what it does for you.

RECOMMENDED DIETARY ALLOWANCES, *National Academy of Sciences, National Research Council, Food and Nutrition Board,* 1980.
The latest findings for minimum daily requirements of nutrients, vitamins, and minerals.

U.S. DEPARTMENT OF AGRICULTURE. *Handbook of the Nutritional Contents of Foods,* 1975.
Complete charts of the nutritive values of an extensive variety of foods. A good book for learning what is in the food you eat.

U.S. DEPARTMENT OF HEALTH, EDUCATION, and WELFARE. *Alcohol and Your Unborn Child,* # (ADM) 78–521, 1978.
Must reading for every pregnant woman. Discusses the latest findings on how alcohol affects the unborn child.

WILLIAMS, PHYLLIS, R.N. *Nourishing Your Unborn Child,* 1974.
A basic book on nutrition which can help during pregnancy. Has a variety of appetizing recipes.

Organizations

INTERNATIONAL CHILDBIRTH EDUCATION ASSOCIATION, INC., P.O. Box 20048, Minneapolis, MN 55420.

LA LECHE LEAGUE, INTERNATIONAL, 9616 Minneapolis Avenue, Franklin Park, IL 60131.

MOTHERS OF TWINS, (national organization) 5402 Amberwood Lane, Rockville, MD 20803.

Pregnancy

BING, ELIZABETH; and COLMAN, LIBBY. *Making Love During Pregnancy,* 1977.
A clear, straightforward, and honest discussion of the interrelationship of pregnancy and sexuality. Well illustrated with beautiful line drawings. Should be required reading for all parents-to-be. Highly recommended.

BREWER, GAIL S. *The Pregnancy after 30 Workbook,* 1978.
A positive approach to childbearing in the thirties. Includes a variety of articles on diet, self-awareness, and exercise for trouble-free birth and post-partum period. Exercise section very limited.

FLANAGAN, GERALDINE, L. *The First Nine Months of Life,* 1962.
An extensively chronicled discussion of the prenatal period. Well illustrated with photos at various stages of development. Recommended.

HOTCHNER, TRACY. *Pregnancy and Childbirth,* 1979.
An encyclopedia on pregnancy, breastfeeding, and postpartum. Good reading for factual information. Organization is lacking.

MONTAGU, ASHLEY. *Life before Birth,* 1977.
An exciting exploration of the prenatal child's world and how the mother affects and interacts with it. Recommended.

Parenting

DODSON, FITZHUGH. *How to Parent,* 1970.
A child psychologist's very practical guide to parenting. Has extensive section on toys, books, and records for various age levels. Highly recommended.

FRAIBERG, SELMA. *The Magic Years,* 1959.
Excellent insight into the interior life of the infant and young child. Highly recommended.

KELLY, MARGUERITE; and PARSON, ELIA. *The Mother's Almanac,* 1975.
A wonderfully thorough and creative book of helpful information on living with small children. Ideas and activities are applied to various levels ages 1–6. Highly recommended.

Rakowitz, Elly; and Rubin, Gloria. *Living with Your New Baby: A Postpartum Guide for Mothers and Fathers,* 1978.
Good description of feelings and situations in early parenthood.

Spock, Benjamin. *Baby and Child Care,* 1978.
The handbook for knowing when to call the doctor if your child is sick. Useful for symptoms of illness and better understanding of your growing. child. Recommended.

Wright and Inmon. *Preparing for Parenthood,* 1980.
Enjoyable and practical book for the postpartum period.

Parenting Magazines

Mothering, P.O. Box 2046; Albuquerque, NM 87103. Subscription: $8.00 per year.
A wonderful and touching magazine with articles written by mothers relating their feelings, experiences, etc. Well worth reading and saving.

Postpartum

Bing, Elizabeth; and Colman, Libby. *Making Love During Pregnancy,* 1977.
See pregnancy section for details.

Pizer, Hank; and Garfink, Christine. *The Postpartum Book: How to Cope with and Enjoy the First Year of Parenting,* 1979.
A realistic yet supportive guide that surveys the feelings and reactions that accompany the arrival of a new baby.

Rozdilsky, Marylou; and Banet, Barbara. *What Now? a Handbook of New Parents Postpartum,* 1975 (Revised).
A straightforward, often funny, guidebook for new parents. Covers information on physical changes after birth, sex, depression, shared responsibilities, etc. Highly recommended.

Relaxation

Benson, Herbert. *The Relaxation Response,* 1975.
Clear, scientific understanding of how to learn to relax.

Hinrichsen, Gerda. *The Body Shop,* 1974.
A noted Danish physiotherapist writes about relieving tension via stretching exercises. Very compatible with hatha yoga practices.

White, John; and Fadiman, James. *Relax: How You Can Feel Better, Reduce Stress and Overcome Tension,* 1976.
Exploration of a variety of approaches for inducing relaxation. Good book for better understanding of the relaxation response.

Index to Asanas

General Index